The
Complete Illustrated
Birthing Companion

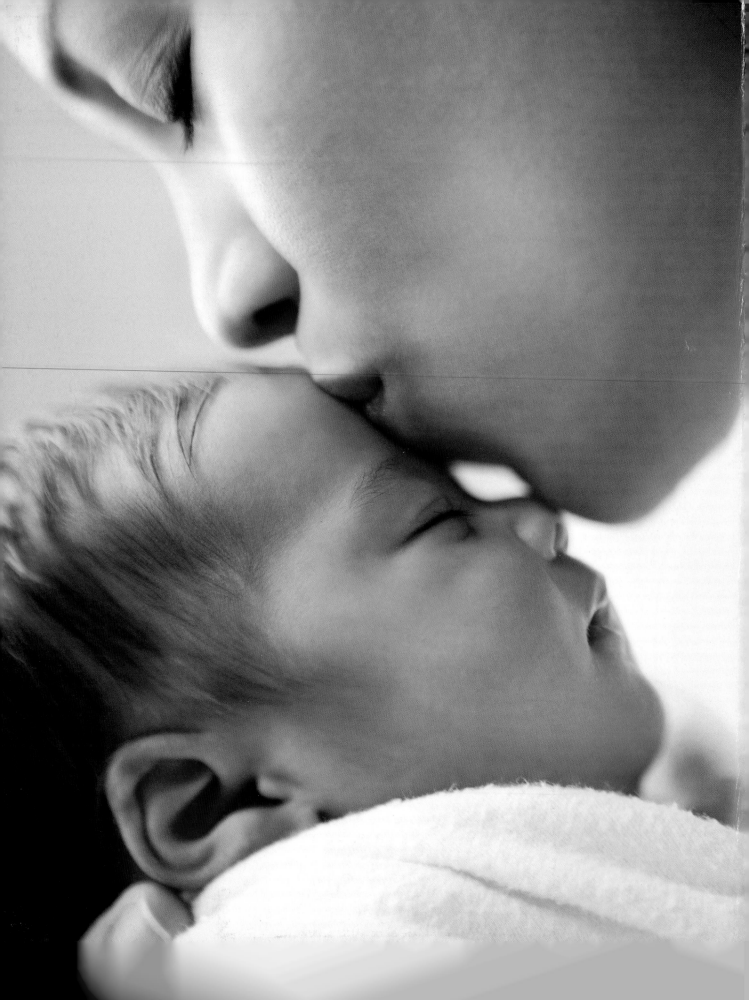

The Complete Illustrated Birthing Companion

A Step-by-Step Guide to Creating the
Best Birthing Plan for a Safe, Less Painful, and
Successful Delivery for You and Your Baby

Amanda V. French, M.D.
Gynecologist, Brigham and Women's Hospital and Boston Children's Hospital
Clinical Instructor of Obstetrics, Gynecology and Reproductive Biology, Harvard Medical School

Susan Thomforde, C.N.M. • **Jeanne Faulkner, R.N.** • **Dana Rousmaniere**

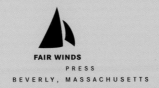

FAIR WINDS
PRESS
BEVERLY, MASSACHUSETTS

Text © 2012 Amanda French, M.D., Susan Thomforde, C.N.M., Jeanne Faulkner, R.N., Dana Rousmaniere

First published in the USA in 2012 by
Fair Winds Press, a member of
Quayside Publishing Group
100 Cummings Center
Suite 406-L
Beverly, MA 01915-6101
www.fairwindspress.com

16 15 14 13 12   1 2 3 4 5

ISBN: 978-1-59233-533-6

Digital edition published in 2012
eISBN: 978-1-61058-624-5

Library of Congress Cataloging-in-Publication Data
The complete illustrated birthing companion: a step-by-step guide to creating the best birthing plan for a safe, less painful, and successful delivery for you and your baby / Amanda V. French ... [et al.].
     p. cm.
  Includes bibliographical references.
  ISBN 978-1-59233-533-6
 1. Childbirth--Popular works. I. French, Amanda V.
  RG651.C62 2012
  618.2--dc23

                    2012020537

Cover and book design by Fair Winds Press
Book layout by Megan Jones Design (www.meganjonesdesign.com)
Illustrations by Judy Love (www.judyloveillustration.com)

Cover images: Shutterstock.com, top, left; iStockphoto.com, middle; Ian Hooten/Science Photo Library/gettyimages.com, right. Back cover images: Goldmund Lukic/gettyimages.com, left; Shutterstock.com, second, left; iStockphoto.com, middle; image 100/agefotostock.com, second, right; Fotolia.com, right

Printed and bound in Singapore

DEDICATION

Thank you to my three fellow authors for asking me to collaborate on this project. I am proud to be a member of the team. I would also like to acknowledge all of the patients I have seen over the years, for they have taught me that there is a difference between answering a question with a quote from a textbook and answering a question in a practical, user-friendly way. Most of all, I would like to thank my family, and especially my husband. His support has helped me make some difficult but wonderful decisions in my life.

—Amanda French

I would like to thank all the hundreds of women I have cared for during my career as a midwife. They have let me into their lives and have taught me to trust the birth process. It is a marvel to watch "my babies" grow up to be wonderful young adults with lives of their own. Infinite thanks go to my husband, who has supported me through the many years of erratic and unpredictable schedules, and to my three wonderful young adult children, who know the ups and downs of having a mom who is a midwife.

—Susan Thomforde

For Jerome whose love, support, and faith mean everything
For my babies—Lauren, Camille, Lee, Olivia, and Lua
For my mother, sharing this with me from beyond
For the women in the world who need our help and the ones who teach us how to be mothers

—Jeanne Faulkner

To Will, who held my hand, massaged my back, got in the tub, stood beside me—and stood behind me—for every one of our births
To Julia, Charlie, and Jack, whose births changed my life
To my own mother, who helped me get back on my feet after each and every delivery and who taught me what it means to be a mom
And to all the women who read this book—may your own baby's birth be a safe and satisfying experience. Congratulations on the journey ahead.

—Dana Rousmaniere

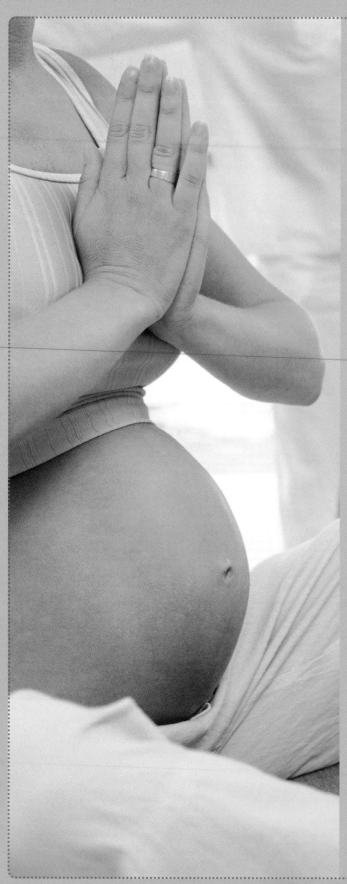

Contents

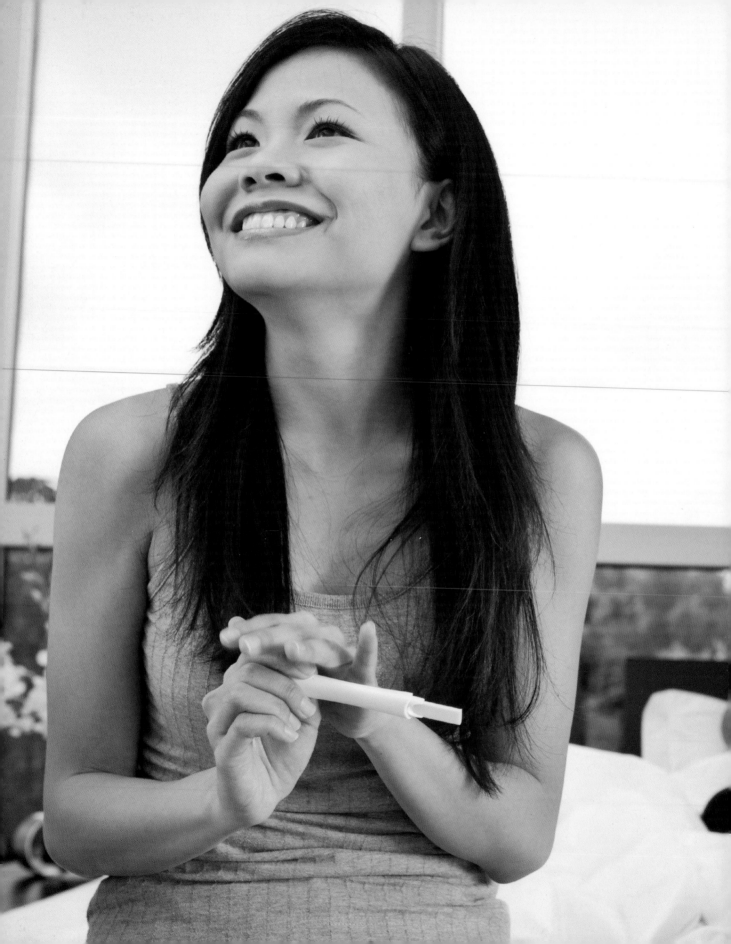

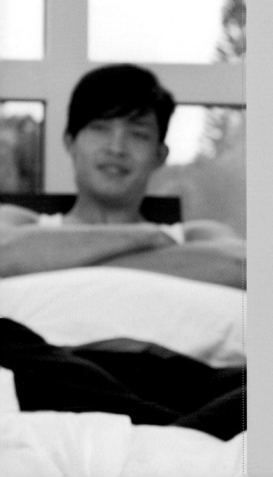

Congratulations— You're Pregnant!

Now what?

What an exciting, awe-inspiring time in your life, filled with the magic and wonder of the tiny life growing inside of you. From the moment you first laid eyes on that positive pregnancy test, you've no doubt been thinking ahead to the day you'll get to meet your little one. Whether this is your first baby or your fourth, you're bound to have tons of questions about what lies ahead. You may be filled with worry, fear, excitement, anxiety, and everything in between. Maybe you're wondering what kind of mother you'll be or how you're going to get through labor and delivery.

Rest assured that you're already doing what's best for you and your baby—educating yourself about what to expect during your baby's birth, so you can have the safest, most satisfying, and most successful delivery. Consider this book your go-to guide for getting there. In the pages ahead, you'll find a comprehensive look at everything you need to know to take the fear and anxiety out of your birth experience. This book will empower you to take charge of your birthing experience, giving you the confidence and conviction that you've put the best possible plan in place for the right birth for you.

Sometimes the best-laid birth plans don't go according to plan. Maybe you've prepared for an all-natural delivery but need to have an emergency Cesarean section. Or maybe you planned to get an epidural, but arrive at the hospital already 10 centimeters dilated, ready to start pushing. That's why this book covers all the options out there—from natural delivery to C-section—from an unbiased viewpoint, presenting you with the information you'll need to prepare yourself for any eventuality. We'll give you an insider's perspective on labor and delivery in our "Real Deal" and "Inside Information" sections, where our labor nurse, Jeanne Faulkner, tells you what really goes on in a labor and delivery room.

The more you equip yourself with information about all the potential options for giving birth, the better prepared you'll be if you suddenly find yourself needing to shift gears at the last minute.

Here's what this book is not: It's not intended to be a comprehensive guide to your pregnancy. Instead we've focused on your baby's birth—because we simply couldn't find a book that adequately prepares women for what to expect in any given birth scenario. So we decided to write it ourselves.

WHO ARE WE?

We're moms like you. It wasn't that long ago that each one of us was reading every pregnancy and birth book we could get our hands on. Collectively we've given birth to twelve children of our own, all in varying styles—from water birth to hospital birth with an epidural.

Amanda French, MD, FACOG, is a board-certified obstetrician and gynecologist who completed her training at Boston Medical Center. She has been employed in both private practice and academic medicine teaching residents and students obstetrics and gynecology at Brigham and Women's Hospital in Boston and Columbia Presbyterian Medical Center in New York City. Currently Dr. French is a pediatric and adolescent gynecologist for Boston Children's Hospital and Brigham and Women's Hospital and a clinical instructor for Harvard Medical School. She has delivered more than 1,000 babies over the course of her career and is the proud mother of two energetic little boys.

Susan Thomforde, CNM, is a practicing certified nurse midwife who trained at the University of Utah. She worked in hospitals for ten years and has spent the past seventeen years delivering babies and providing gynecological care at the North Shore Birth Center in Beverly, Massachusetts—one of only two free-standing birth centers in the state. She's been called "a midwife's midwife"—to her, the highest compliment there is. She has helped train many nurse midwifery students, helping to ensure that midwifery stays alive and well in the United States. Susan's three babies—now wonderful young adults—were delivered by her sister midwives.

Jeanne Faulkner, RN, spent almost twenty years working as a registered nurse in labor and delivery departments in Los Angeles and Portland, Oregon, hospitals. She's still a nurse and has been writing full-time for magazines, newspapers, and websites for ten years. She writes *Fit Pregnancy*'s "Ask the Labor Nurse" column (which won Min-online's Best of the Web, best blog of 2012) and contributes articles about global maternal health and women's issues to the *Huffington Post*. She's also the chairperson for advocacy for CARE (a global humanitarian organization) in Oregon and writes for many publications about the work it does to alleviate poverty. Her children include three daughters, a beloved niece, and one son.

Dana Rousmaniere has written about pregnancy and parenting for years, as managing editor of *Fit Pregnancy* magazine online and for popular pregnancy, parenting, and women's health sites and publications such as *Good Housekeeping*, *Women's Health*, Babble.com, and CaféMom.com. She's also the author of *North Shore Baby*, a field guide for parents living north of Boston. Her first two babies were delivered in a hospital with an OB/GYN and an epidural, and her third—a 10.5-pound (4.76 kg) baby!—was delivered in a drug-free water birth at a birth center.

What Lies Ahead . . .

In the chapters that follow, we'll introduce you to all of your options for giving birth—from traditional to alternative. We'll present the pros and cons of each option and offer helpful tips and tools for deciding on a birth plan that suits you best. We'll talk about what happens when things don't go according to plan, so you'll be prepared for any eventuality on the day of your delivery. We'll walk you through creating your own birth plan—from deciding on

big-picture birthing styles to nailing down specific pain-management techniques. We'll guide you through every step of the way, showing you what to expect, so you'll be more than prepared for the big day. From managing the pain of labor to choosing a health care provider and assembling your birth team, you'll learn all the ins and outs you need to know to have an empowered birth experience.

A NOTE FROM THE AUTHORS

It has been an honor and a pleasure for us to collaborate on this book. Sharing our diverse backgrounds and naturally independent points of view has allowed us to provide you with a comprehensive view of the birthing options available. Our collective wisdom and knowledge provide opinions and viewpoints from all of our unique perspectives, which are all represented in the pages of this book. However, each one of us may not support *all* of the options or viewpoints you read about here.

We appreciate the opportunity to share our varied opinions and viewpoints with you and recognize that everyone's experience is unique. We're proud to advocate for women and empower them to become informed about their choices.

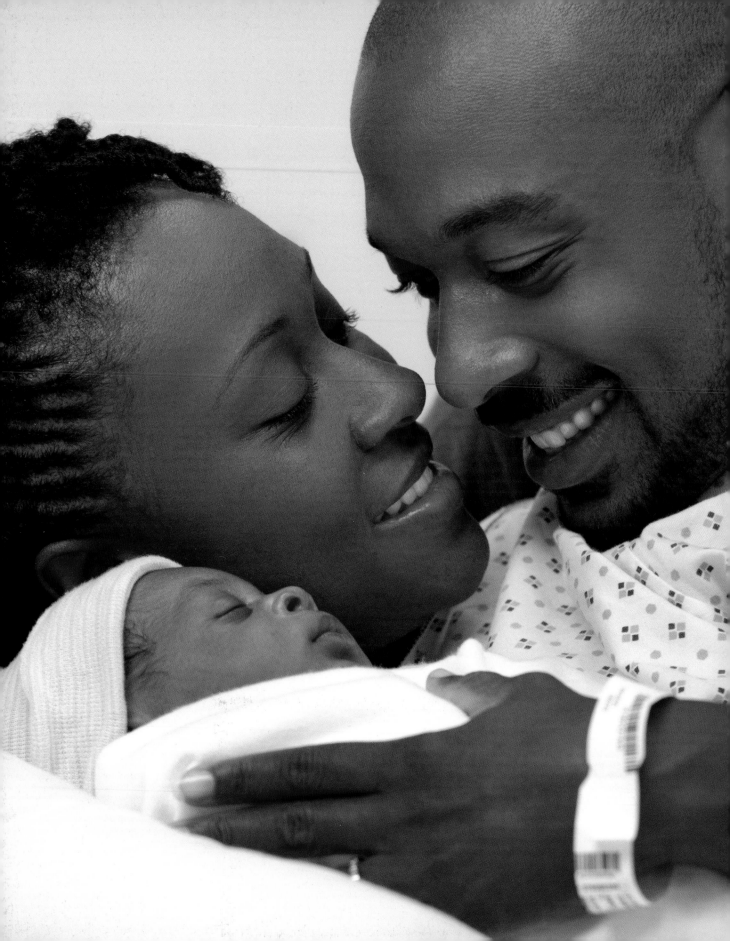

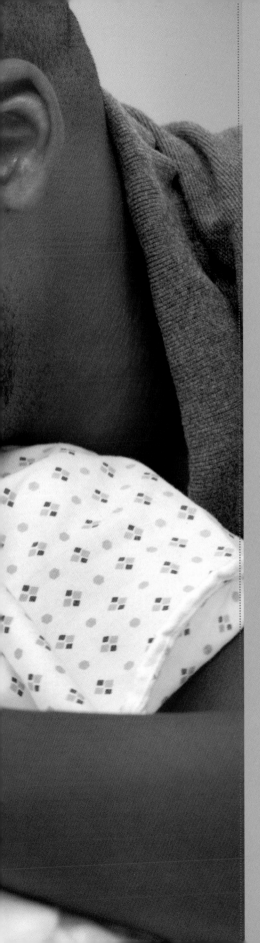

CHAPTER 1

What's Your Birthing Style?

From home birth to high-tech hospital birth

You're going to look back on your baby's birth for years to come, recalling the most minute details of the life-changing day you brought your baby into the world. Maybe you'll document it in a video, photo montage, or "birth story." Someday you'll tell your child all about the day he or she was born.

Close your eyes and think about it: How do you envision your baby's birth? Surely you see your child coming into the world in the safest way possible. But how do you see your baby and yourself in that moment? How are you feeling about your environment and the process of giving birth? Are you in a bed at your local hospital, as your trusted OB/GYN helps your partner cut the baby's cord, with friends and family in the waiting room? Are you in a tub of warm water as a midwife brings your baby to the surface for his first breath of air? Are you in your own home, with the lights dimmed, candles lit, and a doula by your side? Think about your labor. How would you spend the hours leading up to your baby's birth? Are you walking the hospital corridors? Taking a walk on the beach or around your neighborhood? Meditating in a quiet, candlelit room? Relaxing in a hospital bed with the help of an epidural?

Now that you've got an image of your baby's birth in your head, focus on it for a minute and then . . . let it go. Imagine another scenario—maybe one where you're being rushed into an operating room for an emergency C-section, or one where you're having natural childbirth because your labor progressed too quickly for an epidural. Really think about it, because the truth is, no woman can say how her labor and delivery will unfold. Every birth is different, and we all know what can happen to the best-laid plans. (News flash: Babies don't read birth plans!) Sometimes the plan will need to change—in a split second—for the sake of a healthy mom and baby.

That's why we've designed this book to give you an unbiased, realistic understanding of all the ways a birth might unfold. We give it to you straight—the pros and cons of every birth path, and the real reasons why—in collaboration with your trusted caregiver—you may or may not find yourself walking that path.

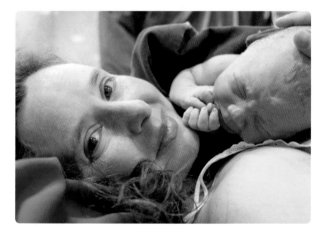

Your perfect birth will be the one in which you're holding your perfect baby in your arms, and mom and baby are safe and sound.

Now put the image of your perfect birth back in your head, and hold on to it. Because right now—by reading this book—you're putting the plans in place to give you the optimal conditions for getting there. Think about your perfect birth and believe that you have the power to bring it about. And in the end, know that however your labor and delivery unfold, your perfect birth will be the one in which you're holding your perfect baby in your arms.

In this chapter, we'll help you begin to lay the groundwork for your baby's birth. Here's where you start imagining the possibilities: It begins with figuring out how you'd ideally like your labor and delivery to unfold. We'll help you think through whether you're leaning toward a natural birth, high-tech help, or some middle road such as a birth center on the grounds of a hospital. We'll help you think through why you may lean toward one option or the other, what to expect in any given birth scenario, and what the pros and cons of each scenario might be. We'll give you an overview of some of the more well-known schools of thought in childbirth education and pain management to help you begin thinking through your own personal philosophy of birth. We'll also help you think through how to find the right health care practitioner for you.

LABOR AND DELIVERY FAQS

The smartest way to approach labor and birth is with curiosity and questions. Here are a few frequently asked questions from first-time and experienced mothers—we'll provide more in-depth information and answers to other questions in the coming chapters.

Q: *How much will labor and birth hurt?*
A: That depends on pain management techniques, how long labor lasts, and other factors, but most women say it's the most painful event of their lives.

Q: *How long will labor last?*
A: First labors average about twelve hours. Subsequent labors usually go quicker.

Q: *Whom should I have with me?*
A: Your husband or partner, mother, sister, friend, doula, and/or anyone else who will truly help you through labor. Don't invite people who can't put your needs first.

Q: *What's the best pain management option?*
A: Pain is subjective, and managing it depends on how you experience it. Some women need only relaxation techniques and a tub of warm water. Others need every drug in the pharmacy. We'll cover all the options in chapter 10.

Q: *Can I do it drug free?*
A: Of course you can. Not so long ago drug free was the only option. We'll cover natural pain management in chapter 10.

Q: *Can I get an epidural right away?*
A: It's not instant, and there are significant advantages to waiting until active labor. We'll cover epidurals in chapter 5.

Q: *Will I tear, poop, pee, or vomit?*
A: Straight up? You might, but there are ways to lower the odds. We'll provide you with tips for managing the unpleasant physiology of childbirth in upcoming chapters.

Q: *Is it safe to deliver at home?*
A: For some women, yes. For others—not so much. Chapter 2 can help you determine whether it's safe for you.

Q: *Will my next labor be quicker than my first?*
A: Most likely, but there's no guarantee.

Q: *What if I deliver in the car?*
A: Consider yourself lucky that your labor was fast. Have your driver pull over and "catch." Keep the umbilical cord attached to both baby and placenta, put the baby skin-to-skin to your breast, wrap blankets or jackets around the two of you, and head to the hospital.

Q: *What if I get to the hospital too late for an epidural?*
A: Again, consider yourself lucky that your labor was quick. Will it hurt? Yes! Will it be over quickly? Yes! Will you be okay? Yes! Women delivered without epidurals for thousands of years. You can, too.

THE REAL DEAL: *A Perfect Birth*

You know that perfect birth you're envisioning? It just might be your second birth, not your first one. That's because first labors usually last longer and hurt more than most women imagine and aren't what they thought they were getting into at all. Even women who say labor isn't painful, "just intense," often hadn't figured it would be quite as "intense" as it really was.

Your body has a learning curve when it comes to having babies. Your uterus has to get organized about how hard and how often to contract. Your cervix has to dilate for the first time, your pelvic bones have to soften and mold, and your vagina has to stretch.

Women sometimes start labor with plans, techniques, and demands for how they want things to play out. When reality hits, however, sometimes those plans just don't cut it. It's especially difficult if labor doesn't proceed smoothly or baby doesn't tolerate labor well. That's why it's wise to also consider contingency plans.

It's the second labor that usually winds up being the dream birth. If first labors are long, then second labors tend to be quick because your body knows what to do. It may not be any less intense, but the intensity doesn't generally last as long as with the first labor. That's why many mothers consider their second birth a much better experience than their first.

Third (fourth, fifth, etc.) births usually progress more quickly than the first, but not necessarily quicker than the second. That may be because the uterus is less toned than it was the first and second time around.

If your first birth doesn't go as planned, you're in good company with millions of other mothers, and you can always use that birth plan for your next baby.

Q: *How can I avoid all those interventions I had with my first labor?*

A: That depends on your individual health factors. We'll talk about routine and special interventions, which ones you need, and which ones you can avoid.

Q: *I had a C-section. Can I have a vaginal birth this time?*

A: Although the American Congress of Obstetricians and Gynecologists (ACOG) is officially supportive of vaginal births after Cesarean births (VBACs), not all hospitals and insurance providers are on board with this position. We'll cover VBACs in chapter 7.

ALL NATURAL, HIGH TECH, OR SOMEWHERE IN BETWEEN?

Planning for birth depends on the style that fits you best: all natural, high tech, or middle ground. Here's a quick rundown of all your options plus their pros and cons to help you choose the best style for you, your baby, and your family.

All Natural

For some women, natural childbirth means no pain medication. For others, it means vaginal delivery. ACOG doesn't have a definition for natural childbirth, instead categorizing birth with more specific terms: vaginal, Cesarean, VBAC, or operative.

"'Natural childbirth' isn't a true medical term," says coauthor Amanda French, MD, OB/GYN. "When a patient tells me she wants to 'go natural,' I ask her, 'what exactly do you have in mind? Usually, she means no pain medicine, but the definition can be rather broad."

"I'd define 'natural birth' as labor experienced without analgesia or regional anesthesia, and birth without instrumental assistance. But women can have local anesthesia and still consider it natural childbirth," says coauthor Susan Thomforde, CNM.

For the purposes of this book, *natural childbirth* means labor without pain medication and vaginal delivery without forceps or vacuum extraction.

'Natural childbirth' isn't a true medical term.

—Amanda French, MD, OB/GYN

Pros and Cons of Natural Childbirth

The most obvious advantage is that a natural, low-intervention, unmedicated vaginal birth can be the safest, healthiest birth option for many mothers and babies. As women all throughout history have given birth naturally, it's a powerful experience that links women of all generations. That's not to say if epidurals were available thousands of years ago, some of our ancestors wouldn't have lined up.

Most natural childbirth techniques are non-invasive, which means there's less chance they'll harm or intrude on mom or baby. Also, mothers can move freely, change positions, and participate actively in their birth experience. It minimizes the need for other medical interventions such as IVs, extensive fetal heart monitoring, and use of drugs such as Pitocin. Fathers and partners participate in active support throughout labor and birth. It can be an exhilarating, empowering, and rewarding life experience.

As for the cons, natural childbirth may not be the healthiest or best option for all women. If labor is more painful, longer, or more challenging than anticipated, and natural techniques aren't adequate, then natural childbirth might not feel empowering and rewarding at all. Instead, having no other pain management option can make some women feel trapped, terrified, and traumatized.

If you've decided to go all natural, you have lots of options and several decisions to make:

Where will you deliver? You can have natural childbirth anywhere, but some women say they feel most supported to have a natural birth at home or in a birth center for the following reasons:

- Hospital-based pain management techniques such as epidurals aren't available.
- They're more likely to be delivered by a midwife with natural childbirth experience.
- There's more access to birthing tubs and freedom to move around during labor.

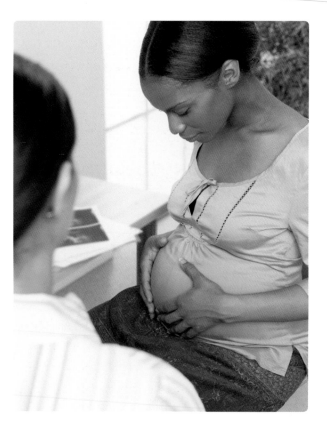

A qualified midwife or doctor can support natural childbirth, but a midwife might be your best choice. Midwives tend to have more experience with natural techniques and view labor and birth as a normal, not medical event.

Who will deliver you? Any qualified midwife or doctor can support natural childbirth, but midwives may be more experienced and supportive of natural births, while doctors may have more experience with medicated or complicated births. Hospital-based midwives may feel more comfortable using medical pain management than midwives who practice at home or birth centers.

Who will support you? Your husband, partner, mother, sister, or friend can be your primary support person if he or she is well prepared. You might consider hiring a doula to do the heavy work of labor support and let your partner and family focus on emotional support. Your labor nurses and midwife will also be part of your support system.

How will you manage labor pain? There are dozens of options ranging from Lamaze to Hypno-Birthing to Orgasmic Birthing to Waterbirth. There's Birthing From Within, the Bradley Method, acupuncture, massage, and countless variations of breathing and relaxation techniques.

The Middle Ground

Maybe you're leaning toward a natural birth but want the option of advanced medical help. Maybe you've decided home birth isn't for you, but you don't want a traditional hospital experience either. Maybe you're not sure what you want. You might choose one of these middle ground options: a freestanding birth center located in or near a hospital or a hospital birth with a doctor or midwife who's supportive of natural birth, but one who can also switch gears quickly if necessary.

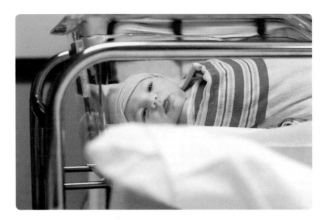

Most babies are born healthy and won't need intensive medical care. Not every maternity unit has a NICU, but all have the ability to transfer sick babies to a hospital that does.

Pros

- You have a full range of birth options available.
- Emergency help is immediately available.
- If you want an epidural, it's available.
- If your baby needs special care in the nursery, it's right there.

Note: Not every hospital that has a maternity unit has a neonatal intensive care unit, but it will have the ability to transfer a baby who needs the NICU to a hospital that has one.

Cons

Hospital-based birth centers follow many of the same standards of care as hospitals, which might include more restrictions and interventions than you want. Also, the temptation to use pain medication might be increased because it's easier to get in a hospital birth center.

High-Tech Help

Some women have health factors that mean the hospital is absolutely the best place for them to deliver. About 300,000 women die in childbirth every year. Though most of those women are in developing countries, women also die in the United States, Europe, and other societies with easy-to-access health care. Certainly some women die in hospitals, too, but many women who might otherwise be seriously injured in childbirth deliver safely and take home a healthy baby because they have access to skilled, hospital-based, medical expertise.

For many women, the hospital is the only place to give birth because they want the following:

- Narcotic and epidural pain management
- Doctors, midwives, and nurses to take care of them
- A couple of days to rest after birth
- Access to breastfeeding consultants, postpartum and nursery nurses, pediatricians, and other specialists
- Their own personal space to deliver, recover, and rest in relative privacy because they have other children or family members at home

Pros

Hospital births provide all medical services, including anesthesia and intensive care. New mothers receive housekeeping, room service, and round-the-clock nursing care. They also get their own personal space (away from the demands of home) to deliver and recover.

Cons

Hospitals can have strict rules and standards that might feel inflexible to some families. Also, they're not home or comfortable for everyone.

AN OVERVIEW OF SOME POPULAR BIRTHING SCHOOLS OF THOUGHT

HypnoBirthing, also known as the Mongan Method, uses the principles of self-hypnosis to help a woman enter a state of deep relaxation during childbirth. The idea is not that you'll be in a "trance" for your delivery but rather that you'll be fully alert, present, and calm. HypnoBirthing relies on tools such as visualization, affirmations, and the power of suggestion to train women to let go of the fear associated with natural childbirth—thereby releasing the pain that can come from tensing your body in fear. The underlying philosophy is that if you can completely trust your body and your natural birthing instincts, you can let go of the fear/pain cycle and have a calm, centered birth experience.

But does it work? HypnoBirthing's self-reported statistics claim that only 23 percent of mothers birthing vaginally had epidural anesthesia, compared with the national average of 71 percent, and that from 2005 to 2010, 17 percent of U.S. HypnoBirthing mothers birthed via C-section, compared with the national average of 32 percent. Our take: If you want to give birth naturally, it's one of several good tools to have in your toolbox.

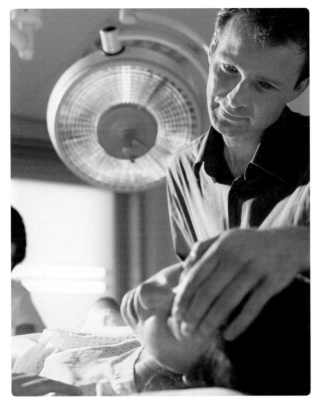

HypnoBirthing trains women to let go of fear and release the pain that comes with tension. This can facilitate a calm, centered birth.

The Bradley Method bills itself as "husband-coached natural childbirth." The prenatal education classes are designed for small groups, and they last an intensive twelve weeks. (That means that if you're thinking of trying the Bradley Method, you should start looking into prenatal classes in your first trimester—don't wait until your third trimester to start.) The Bradley Method teaches couples to work with their bodies to reduce pain and make their labors more efficient. (Its self-reported statistics are impressive, as it claims that "of over 1,000,000 couples trained in the Bradley Method nationwide, over 86 percent of them have had

spontaneous, unmedicated vaginal births.") What you can expect: a lot of reading materials, a big focus on training your labor coach to help you get through labor, and a comprehensive education on prenatal nutrition, fitness, and labor and delivery techniques. Our take: The Bradley Method requires a solid commitment both to the classes and to natural childbirth, as it's a very intensive program. If you're sure you want to give birth naturally, the Bradley Method will teach you some excellent skills. However, some women may find it to be very dogmatic. And some health care practitioners disagree with the "husband-coached" method of childbirth that the Bradley Method teaches, in that it may put too much emphasis on the father's role in childbirth and not enough on the laboring mother's (and her health care provider's). Some women and health care providers simply prefer to have dad in more of an "emotional support" role, rather than an "in charge" role.

So many of us associate **Lamaze** with the "hoo-hoo-hee-hee" method of breathing we've seen from laboring women on TV and in the movies. But Lamaze is about more than just the breathing. Lamaze believes in supporting a natural, healthy, and safe approach to childbirth through education and advocacy. In Lamaze classes you'll learn about healthy birth practices such as letting labor begin on its own, changing positions during labor, avoiding unnecessary interventions, having a labor coach, and bonding immediately with your baby. Our view is that it can provide a good, comprehensive overview of childbirth.

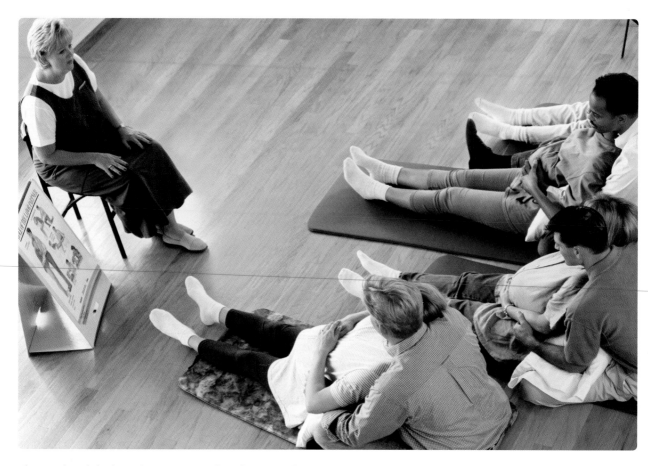

Choosing the right birthing education program depends on you and your partner's personal needs, goals, philosophies, time frame, and what's available in your area.

Birthing From Within's mission is to inspire and teach expecting parents (and those who work with them) to prepare for birth as a rite of passage (and not as a medical event); to understand the power and lifelong impact of birthing from within; to prevent or minimize emotionally difficult births; and to create holistic prenatal care. Birthing From Within classes teach women that the essence of childbirth preparation is self-discovery, not learning obstetric information. Class content is determined by parents' individual needs, and classes don't focus on a specific birth outcome but rather on "preparing women to give birth-in-awareness." Birthing From Within advocates that parents deserve support for any birth option that might be right for them (whether that means drugs, C-section, home birth, etc.). They also believe that fathers and birth partners help best as "birth guardians or loving partners" and not as coaches, because they also need support. Our take: We really like *Birthing From Within*. It happens to be coauthor Susan Thomforde's favorite birthing book.

Which "Birthing School" Is Right for Me?

All of the birthing schools of thought described here will help you lay the groundwork for a safe, natural childbirth experience. It all comes down to which method suits your own personal needs and preferences. See what's offered in your local area. Determine how much time you have to commit to any given class. (For instance, if you and your partner don't have twelve weeks, don't sign up for the Bradley Method.)

And think about whether you lean more toward an inwardly focused childbirth experience (e.g., HypnoBirthing) or a more team-focused childbirth experience (e.g., the Bradley Method or Lamaze). Also think about whether you want to focus more on giving birth from a philosophical standpoint (e.g., Birthing From Within) or whether you'd like to gain more technical knowledge about the process of giving birth (e.g., Lamaze).

CHOOSING YOUR HEALTH CARE PROVIDER

Selecting the right person to deliver your baby can make all the difference to your birth experience. Even if you live in an area where your choices are limited, you can still influence your labor and birth by becoming educated on all your options.

Here's a rundown of the different health care providers and their delivery styles.

Midwives are becoming an increasingly popular choice for home, birth center, and hospital births because their philosophy, practice style, and affordability attracts a lot of families. The Midwife's Model of Care is based on pregnancy and birth as normal life events for most women. But "midwife" isn't a one-size-fits-all title. There are several different types with distinct certifications, licenses, education, and training backgrounds. Anybody can call herself a midwife. Make sure she has excellent training, experience, and credentials.

Certified nurse-midwives (CNMs) are registered nurses who've graduated from an accredited nurse-midwifery education program and passed a national certification examination. CNMs practice legally in hospitals, birth centers, and private homes in all fifty states.

Certified midwives (CMs) come from health backgrounds other than nursing, graduate from an accredited midwifery education program, and take the same national certification examination as CNMs. CMs practice legally in several states (including New York, New Jersey, and Rhode Island).

Certified professional midwives (CPMs) meet standards for certification by the North American Registry of Midwives. This is the only midwifery credential that requires expertise in out-of-hospital settings. CPMs practice in private homes and freestanding birth centers.

Direct entry midwives are educated either through self-study, apprenticeship, midwifery school, or college/university-based programs that don't include nursing. Many CMs and CPMs are direct entry midwives.

Lay midwives are educated through self-study and/or apprenticeships. Many are highly skilled and experienced but aren't certified or licensed.

What kind of midwife should you choose? If you're planning a hospital birth, you'll need a certified nurse midwife. Home birth or birth center? All types of midwives are excellent choices.

Naturopaths (NDs) are doctors of naturopathic medicine. They study all the same sciences as medical doctors (MDs), plus holistic and nontoxic therapies, including nutrition, acupuncture,

Inside Information

If yours is a high-intervention pregnancy (even if it's not particularly high risk), you might wind up with a high-intervention labor. There are countless tests, procedures, and interventions you can choose or opt out of during pregnancy. Though some are important for all pregnant women, others are entirely optional. Not every mother needs an ultrasound, though some need several. Not every family wants genetic testing, though it's highly recommended for many. Not every mother needs every test on the menu, though many opt for the full-meal deal, just in case.

Many women start pregnancy intending to have a low-intervention, natural birth, but then slide into a high-intervention pregnancy. Maybe they opt for advanced testing because they're curious or anxious and feel reassured all possible details are covered. Or maybe unforeseen complications come up that change the type of prenatal care they need.

Women who feel more comfortable with increased testing, screening, and medical scrutiny during pregnancy might not feel secure during labor without more of the same.

If you're a low-risk woman who wants a natural birth, choose health care providers who won't insist on nonessential tests and interventions. On the other hand, if you're a high-risk mother with health complications, it makes sense to choose providers who do closer monitoring and more advanced testing.

When your provider recommends prenatal tests and interventions, ask the following questions:

- What are they for and why do you need them?
- How might the results affect your pregnancy and care?
- Are they mandatory or optional?
- How accurate are the tests? What are the chances of false positive or false negative results?

If they're not essential (and many aren't) and won't change anything, then think about whether you really want that test.

homeopathic medicine, and psychology. Currently NDs can be licensed as primary care general practice physicians in seventeen states. Some NDs complete two years of additional training in midwifery and deliver babies. NDs can't deliver in hospitals, but some deliver in private homes and birth centers.

There are four traditional types of doctors who deliver babies:

Medical doctors (MDs) are the traditional physicians who people think of when they hear the word *doctor*. They complete four years of medical school followed by a specialized residency training program of three to five years in their field.

Doctors of osteopathy (DOs) have all the same medical privileges as medical doctors and practice the full scope of Western medicines. DOs can choose any specialty, prescribe drugs, perform surgeries, and practice medicine anywhere in the United States. Many specialize in obstetrics and deliver in hospitals.

Family practice doctors are medical doctors or doctors of osteopathy who treat patients of all ages. Some also deliver babies. They aren't obstetric specialists, however, and if complications arise, they'll refer to or consult with an obstetrician.

Obstetricians (OBs) are either MDs or DOs with special training in prenatal care, labor, birth, high-risk pregnancy, and surgery. OBs take care of healthy women and patients with medical problems or those at high risk for developing complications. Board-certified OBs pass an initial examination, then an ongoing series of exams throughout their career, given by the American Board of Obstetrics and Gynecology.

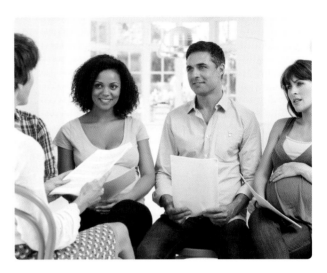

There are many factors to consider when choosing your birthing style such as your family history and birthing background, whether you have had other children, and, of course, your partner's preferences.

Special Considerations When Choosing a Practitioner

Just because they're doctors, it doesn't automatically mean they treat all their patients as potentially sick. In fact, many doctors practice like midwives, respecting the fact that most women are healthy.

Just because they're midwives, it doesn't mean they're experts at natural birth. Many CNMs are trained only in hospitals and use as many medical interventions as any doctor.

Two of the biggest influences that affect almost every health care provider are lawsuits and insurance. Doctors tend to have higher-risk patients and higher malpractice insurance policy premiums than midwives. Doctors and midwives might get sued if something happens to their patient or her baby. Whether it's their fault, or not, they have to be on guard and ready to defend themselves. That can sometimes be why some doctors (and midwives) use interventions to demonstrate they did every-thing possible to diagnose problems and prevent harm to mom and baby.

Defensive medicine can be both a good and a bad policy. Unexpected complications come up in pregnancy, even for the healthiest women. It's reassuring for many women to know their doctor is trained to recognize those possibilities. But other women resent being treated like potential health problems. They prefer to be seen as normal, healthy, and fine. It's a difference in perspective, but not always a big difference in practice styles.

There's a lot to consider when making an in-formed decision about the right doctor or midwife. Do your homework:

- Check out which providers, birth centers, and hospitals are available in your area.
- Ask friends, family, and your primary care phy-sician for recommendations.
- Interview several providers to get a feel for their style, philosophy, practice, and how well they communicate.
- Then ask yourself the following questions:
  - Is this provider the best choice to sup-port my health, pregnancy, birth plan, and family?
  - Is she skilled, easy to access, and does she fit well with my personality?
  - Does she deliver in a location that I'm comfortable with?
  - Can I afford her or does my insurance cover her?

HOW TO MAKE INFORMED CHOICES

What if you're on the fence? If you're leaning toward one birth style but aren't sure if it's right for you, your answers to the following questions could affect your decision-making process.

1. **What's your birthing background?** Virtually every woman has some idea about how birth should be—about how, where, and with whom they want to give birth. Maybe you've grown up in a family of doctors. Maybe you spent your first weeks in a NICU or were born at home. Maybe you admired your sister's Hypno-Birthing techniques or heard a lecture about home-birthing options. Maybe it was a book or newscast that framed the way you think about birth. Evaluate how your history has influenced your birth goals.

2. **Have you had other children?** First births can have a huge effect on subsequent birth choices. Say, for example, you developed complica-tions and had an emergency C-section. Or you wanted a natural birth but felt bullied to use unwanted interventions. Maybe you planned to go all natural but couldn't manage the pain and asked for an epidural. Or maybe everything was perfect. Which elements of your first birth do you want to repeat and which do you want to change?

3. **How have the women in your family given birth?** Though you shouldn't expect to inherit your family's birthing style, certain physical, emotional, and intellectual factors are passed between family members. Will yours be the

first home birth in a hundred years? Have all of your sisters had C-sections? Think about your family's birth legacy as you create your own.

4. **Are there any big differences between your birth plans and your husband's/partner's and family's?** Many people might have strong opinions about what's best for you, but only a few perspectives are crucial: yours, your partner's, and your health care provider's. Your baby's father (or your partner) has a right to feel his child and wife will be safe and well taken care of. If his birth plans are radically different from yours, consider a compromise and counseling to settle on a middle ground. What about the rest of the family? Educate, reassure, and respect them, then proceed with your own decisions.

5. **What's your birth philosophy/dream birth?** The way you envision your perfect birth will influence how you proceed in choosing a provider and birth location. Do you consider birth a medical event or a normal physiologic event? Are you into natural health practices or standard Western medicine? Do you see yourself surrounded by highly skilled doctors and nurses in a hospital or by family and midwives in your own bedroom? No matter what type of birth you've dreamed of, the most important factors to consider are your body type, health history, and current health status. No matter what you hope for, some factors can't be changed. For example, let's say you're five feet (1.5 m) tall, your husband is 6 feet, 5 inches (1.65 m), and

your baby is measuring extremely large for dates. Or maybe you're diabetic, have high blood pressure, or you're carrying triplets. All of these examples describe women at high risk for birth complications and illustrate how risk factors affect your birth choices.

6. **What are your risk factors?**

- **Low risk:** If you're completely healthy and have no health conditions that could affect your delivery (that's most women, by the way), then anything goes. You can choose from the whole menu of birth options from home to hospital, midwife to obstetrician.

- **Medium risk:** If you're basically healthy, but have a couple of variables (such as your age or your weight), you still have lots of options but may want to stick closer to a hospital or birth center.

- **High risk:** Women with specific health concerns should lean toward hospital-based birth options. An obstetrician might be a better choice than a midwife.

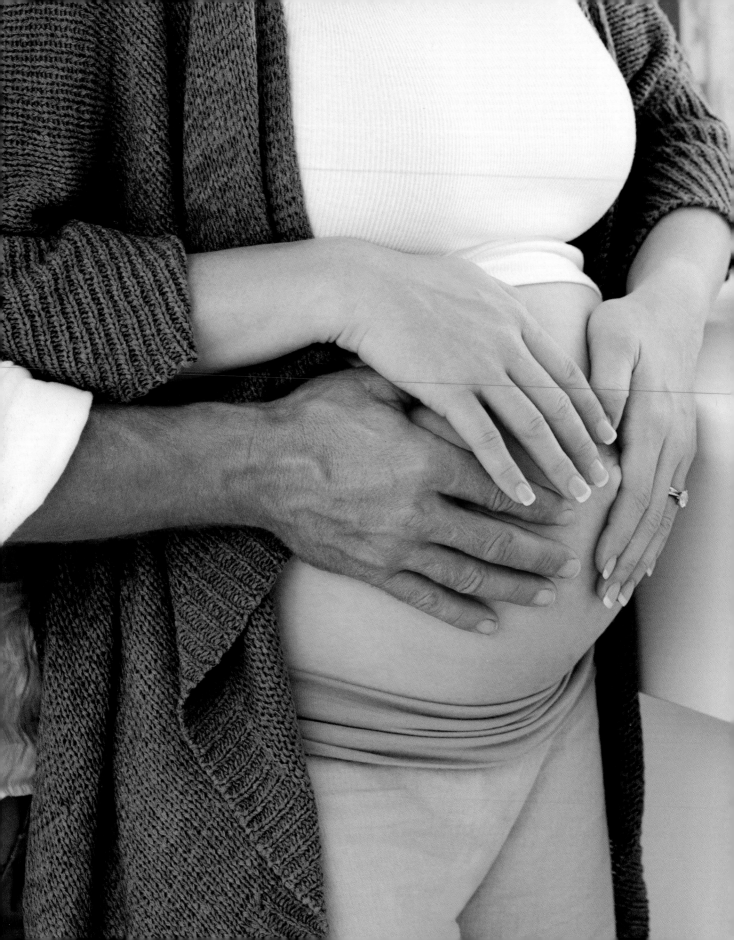

Unmedicated, Vaginal Birth at Home

What it is, why it may or may not be right for you, pros and cons, and how to prepare for this labor path

Unmedicated, vaginal birth at home, also known as home birth, sounds like a fringe option for many women delivering babies in the United States today. The truth is, home birth has been the norm for birthing mothers around the world for most of human history, and it continues to be in many countries and cultures. Giving birth in a hospital is a fairly recent phenomenon. Consider the following statistics from just a few generations ago:

PERCENTAGE OF BIRTHS OCCURRING AT HOME

United States	United Kingdom	Japan
50 percent in 1938	80 percent in the 1920s	95 percent in 1950
1 percent in 1955	1 percent in 1991	1.2 percent in 1975

Source: Tina Cassidy. *Birth*. New York: Atlantic Montly Press, 2006.

It's only in the past century that hospital births have become the norm. This may be in part because of increased access to medical care in developed countries, advances in transportation and medical technology, and the shift from an agricultural to an industrialized society. However, some credit this trend to the rise of private insurance companies in the United States and taxpayer-funded medical care in countries outside the United States, where policies were established that required women to give birth in hospitals.

Though the rate of home birth in the United States is still very low (0.90 percent of births in 2005 and 2006), experts are beginning to see it rise. Home births increased by 5 percent from 2005 and remained steady in 2006, according to the Centers for Disease Control and Prevention (CDC).

WHY HOME BIRTH?

More women are making the choice to give birth in their own homes. Though their reasons vary, for many women, the choice to give birth at home is about reclaiming the birth experience for themselves and their families—approaching it as a normal, natural, instinctive rite of passage rather than as a "medical condition" that necessitates a trip to the hospital. Many women who choose home birth believe that their bodies—and their babies—instinctively know how to give birth and that medical intervention might actually do more harm than good. Other women choose it because they simply want to feel safe and comfortable in their own surroundings and want a more intimate experience.

There are many other reasons why a woman might choose a home birth. Here are a few examples:

- A desire to have more control over what happens during the birth, specifically the following:
  - Fewer vaginal exams
  - Fewer medical interventions such as rupturing the amniotic sac (breaking the water), administering Pitocin to speed up labor or drugs to manage pain, using vacuum extraction and forceps to assist birth, and so on.
  - A desire not to have an IV inserted for labor and delivery
  - No continuous fetal monitoring (A woman giving birth at home with the assistance of a health care provider might expect more intermittent monitoring of mom's and baby's vital signs. For instance, your health care provider might periodically check your blood pressure, pulse, temperature, and your baby's heart rate.)
  - More freedom to choose what you want to wear, eat, and drink, and to move around as you desire
  - More control over who will be present at baby's birth
  - More control over how both mom and baby will spend the first hours and days after giving birth
  - A history of quick labors, which may make a woman want to prepare ahead of time for delivering at home

THE REAL DEAL: *Think Carefully about Whom to Invite to the Birth*

Many mothers who deliver at home say they were unprepared for the "house party" atmosphere that accompanied their birth and postpartum period. One advantage of having your baby at home is that you can have anyone you want at your birth. You can include your family, your friends, and your older children. That's great for some women, but for others, labor isn't the party they thought it would be.

Despite our growing cultural trend toward all-inclusive, family oriented births, many women discover that birth is a far more intense, intimate, and private experience than they'd expected. She might not want the excitement and stimulation that having a crowd invites. She might feel shy about being seen naked. People might not leave when she needs them to, and others might show up that she wasn't expecting. Older children might become anxious, upset, or frightened. Mom might feel too exhausted to party with her crowd, or they might leave a mess she's not prepared to clean up. Whatever the reason, many women find that birth isn't really meant to be a birthday party.

Be careful about whom you invite to attend your home birth. Tell people that you reserve the right to rescind your invitation at any time for any reason. Create guidelines for how long visitors can stay and what to do if you need to clear the room quickly. Make arrangements for children to be cared for by someone other than you or your partner. Make sure someone's assigned to deal with "problem visitors" or those who have strong objections to the homebirth. Make sure mom has private space (like her own bedroom) and a door to close in case she needs privacy. Provide resting space for your midwife, too.

As a general rule, opt for fewer people at your birth. You can always invite guests to visit after delivery when you and your baby are more rested.

- A desire for a lower-cost option for giving birth (especially if you have no health insurance)
- Lack of transportation, for instance, in certain rural areas

The top five reasons women chose home birth were safety, avoidance of unnecessary medical interventions, previous negative hospital experience, more control, and having a more comfortable and familiar environment, according to a study in the March–April 2009 *Journal of Midwifery and Women's Health*.

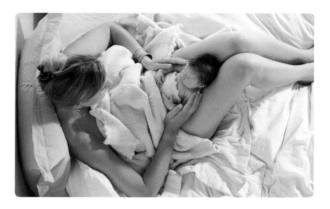

Home birth allows a woman to have a natural birth experience in her own surroundings where she feels most comfortable and supported.

HOW HOME BIRTH DIFFERS FROM A HOSPITAL BIRTH

If you're planning an attended homebirth—meaning that your birth will be attended by a health care provider, usually a midwife or a layperson trained in managing homebirths—your health care provider will still want to see you for regular prenatal care during your pregnancy—these visits might happen in your home rather than an office.

The most obvious difference in the birth experience will be when you actually go into labor. When that time comes, you'll be able to stay in the comfort of your own home, with the midwife coming to you, rather than you going to the midwife. That means that you'll have a lot more control over your immediate environment. You can surround yourself with your own creature comforts. You can deliver in your own bed if you'd like (keep in mind that it will be messy, and that you'll want to make certain

preparations, which we discuss later in this chapter). You can light candles (often not permitted in hospitals), keep the lights dimmed, or maintain a peaceful and quiet atmosphere (which can be difficult to do in a busy hospital).

But home birth is about more than just being in your own home. There are substantial differences to keep in mind.

THE REAL DEAL: *Coverage*

It costs much less to deliver at home, but unfortunately insurance does not usually cover it, except in a few states such as Vermont and New Hampshire.

Pros

- Lower cost, about 60 percent less, according to the American Pregnancy Association
- More control over your surroundings, and who will be present at your baby's birth
- More immediate and continuous bonding with baby, which can also facilitate breastfeeding

Cons

- If something goes wrong during your labor and delivery (which can happen with little to no warning), you would need to be transferred to a hospital, which can take precious time and delay treatment, thereby putting you and your baby at risk. (See our list of reasons why you may need to be transferred to a hospital.)
- There's double to triple the risk of an infant dying in a planned home birth versus a hospital birth, according to the Mayo Clinic. Granted, the overall risk of an infant dying is very low in either scenario, but it may be a risk that some mothers are simply unwilling to take.
- You won't have the benefit of immediate medical care, a NICU, hospital staff, certain medical equipment, or a nursery to help you take care of yourself and your baby during delivery and in the first few hours and days after giving birth. (However, you can plan to have in-home help via a certified midwife, doula, visiting nurse, or friends and family.)

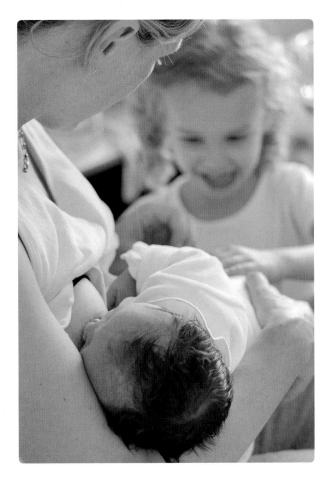

Home birth gives a woman control over who is present at her birth, including her other children, if she and her partner wish. Make sure someone is assigned to care for children during that time and until well after baby is born.

The American Congress of Obstetricians and Gynecologists on Planned Home Births

The American Congress of Obstetricians and Gynecologists (ACOG) issued an official opinion on home birth in February 2011, which says that "although the absolute risk of planned home births is low, published medical evidence shows it does carry a two- to three-fold increase in the risk of newborn death compared with planned hospital births. A review of the data also found that planned home births among low-risk women are associated with fewer medical interventions than planned hospital births."

In a nutshell, ACOG does not support home births. The congress cautions that women who decide to have a home birth should do the following:

- Consider whether they are healthy and "low-risk"
- Work with a certified nurse midwife, certified midwife, or physician who practices in an integrated and regulated health system
- Have ready access to prenatal care
- Have a plan in place for safe and quick transportation to the nearest hospital in the event of an emergency

In contrast, the World Health Organization, the American College of Nurse Midwives, and the American Public Health Association all support home and out-of-hospital birth options for low-risk expectant women.

So Is It Safe?

The safety of home birth is a topic of serious debate. Several studies have argued that for women with normal, healthy pregnancies, home birth is as safe as giving birth in a hospital or birth center. For example, a 1996 study done by a team in Zurich concluded that "for women with low-risk pregnancies in the Netherlands, choosing to give birth at home is a safe choice with an outcome that is at least as good as that of planned hospital birth."

The study also found indications that "there is some self-selection among women who can decide for themselves where to have their baby, and that this preordains outcome, albeit to a limited extent. It is important, therefore, that the home birth option remains available, but especially that women at low risk are really given a free choice."

The study also found that "interventions (induction, Caesarean section, medication, forceps, or vacuum extraction) may be considerably less frequent in women who originally opt for home delivery." More studies are needed to look into the small risks of death, serious bleeding, and other complications that can occur during a home birth, the authors said.

A Real Deal note from our coauthor Dr. Amanda French: "Please keep in mind that you cannot directly compare home births in different countries. The health care systems in the United States and the Netherlands are very different. For example, in the United States, your home could be located hours away from a hospital, and transportation may be very limited. These variables are important in case of an emergency."

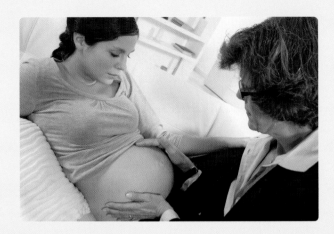

Although ACOG doesn't support home birth, the World Health Organization, American College of Nurse Midwives, and American Public Health Association all advocate home birth for low-risk women.

A 2009 study of 529,688 low-risk planned home and hospital births reported in the *British Journal of Obstetrics and Gynaecology* came to a similar conclusion: "A home birth does not increase the risks of perinatal mortality and severe perinatal morbidity among low-risk women, provided the maternity care system facilitates this choice through the availability of well-trained midwives and through a good transportation and referral system."

Dr. Amanda French: "In the U.S., there is often a lack of a 'referral system' from midwives who do home births to a hospital. Most doctors, in this age of litigation, will not cover home births. Therefore, many midwives who attend home births do not have any official relationship with any hospital."

In the CDC National Vital Statistics Report titled *Trends and Characteristics of Home and Other Out-of-Hospital Births in the United States, 1990–2006*, researchers concluded that "home births were less likely than hospital births to be preterm, low birth weight or multiple deliveries." This is likely because women whose pregnancies are more high risk are delivering in hospitals, while more low-risk women deliver at home. However, the CDC report does say that "because the home birth category contains both planned home births and unplanned home births due to an emergency situation (e.g., a precipitous labor where the mother could not get to the hospital in time), it is unlikely that higher-risk, low-birth-weight, preterm, and multiple births can be completely eliminated from the home birth category."

Other studies have found a higher infant mortality rate in home births as compared with hospital births. Physician groups such as the American Medical Association and ACOG argue that even a normal, healthy birth can have unforeseen complications, and that a medical emergency could happen without warning, thereby making home birth an unsafe option for anyone.

Amanda French, MD: A Physician's View of Home Birth

My personal position on home birth is in line with the American Congress of Gynecologists' Committee Opinion from February 2011. I believe that a hospital or a birthing center with immediate access to a hospital is the safest place to deliver your baby. However, I do agree that women have the right to make their own medical decisions, including choosing their delivery setting, as long as they clearly understand both the benefits and the risks involved. If you came to my office and asked me whether I thought having your baby at home was safe, I would say no. I recommend that you deliver in a hospital. But this is America, and you can do what you want! Part of my job as a physician is to make sure you fully understand the choices you are making.

Who Should Avoid Home Births

There's little debate about the fact that home birth is clearly not a safe idea for certain women. A home birth is probably contraindicated if:

- You have a history of a chronic medical condition, such as diabetes, high blood pressure, or a seizure disorder.
- You are pregnant with multiples.
- You've had a previous C-section.
- You use illegal drugs.
- You develop complications during your pregnancy, such as preeclampsia, gestational diabetes, anemia, or preterm labor.
- Your baby is malpositioned for birth.
- You deliver before 37 weeks or after 42 weeks.

PRENATAL CARE AND PAIN MANAGEMENT FOR HOME BIRTHS

Prenatal care is important for all women. Your health care provider will want to see you regularly and want to discuss the game plan for your home birth, presenting all the "if/then" scenarios for how he or she would handle challenges that may come up during delivery and how they might be addressed differently if you were to deliver in a hospital.

What's home birth without pain medication like? That depends on how you experience pain, how you prepare for labor, how comfortable you feel at home, and which tools you choose to use. It also depends on where you live, because midwives in many countries outside the United States have access to tools American midwives usually don't (such as nitrous oxide and narcotics).

THE REAL DEAL: *Labor Risk*

If you are considered "morbidly obese," preliminary research is beginning to show a threefold increase in late fetal demise. It's a growing problem in the United States, and one that people don't like to hear about, but unfortunately—while the jury is still out and more studies need to be done—it is becoming clear that this is a real health risk.

The way you experience pain is highly subjective, based on an intricate system between your musculoskeletal and nervous system, your brain, and the rest of your body. When your uterus tightens in a strong contraction, muscle tissues communicate with your sensory-nervous system to send a message to the pain center in your brain. Contractions may register as pain very differently in different women. Although most women say contractions during active labor are very painful (ranging between 7 and 10 on a 10-point pain scale), some say they're only mildly painful, uncomfortable, or they feel like very intense pressure.

Some studies say that women who labor at home are well supported, well prepared, and more

Inside Information

Contrary to what some doctors and organizations say, home births are frequently a very safe option for healthy mothers attended by trained, skilled birth attendants. Approximately 1 percent of women deliver at home in the United States, (though home birth rates increased by 20 percent between 2004 and 2008) and most result in safe deliveries. The majority of maternal/newborn complications occur in hospitals. In other countries, a higher percentage of women deliver at home safely. In undeveloped countries where medical care is unavailable and sanitary conditions are poor, there's a higher percentage of complications, but most women still deliver safely at home.

The American Congress of Obstetricians and Gynecologists and the American Medical Association object to home births and say the safest place to deliver is in a hospital or hospital-based birth center. Why are they giving home birth such a bad rap? Because emergencies can and do happen, and sometimes very rapidly. They believe the hospital provides the best odds for being able to delivery quickly and meet mom and baby's emergency needs.

Doctors and hospitals are usually only involved with home birth when something goes wrong. Ask any obstetrician about her home birth experience and she'll most likely remember the patient who stayed home too long with a serious emergency. Maybe the baby survived and maybe she didn't, but the doctor was the one who handled the emergency and was responsible for the patients. This can create a climate of distrust between doctors and midwives and a bias against home births. It's even worse if that family sues the doctor for their mother's or baby's poor outcome. Doctors don't usually see the home births that turn out well. They aren't attending the beautiful deliveries where everyone is healthy and happy, though that's what happens at most home births.

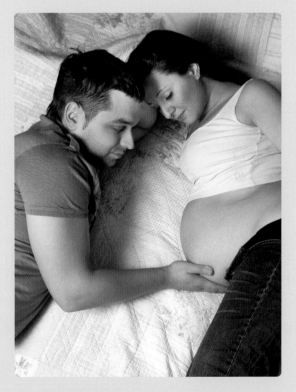

Home births are a safe option for healthy mothers, but emergencies do occur. Doctors don't often see the results of safe home births. They see the emergency cases and therefore, many doctors have strong opinions against the home birth alternative.

relaxed than women in a hospital setting. Relaxation and stress reduction are associated with feeling less pain, but may not be the case for every woman attempting a home birth. Most women say their home birth experience was more comfortable and less painful than a hospital birth.

Women who prepare for labor by becoming well educated about the process of labor and childbirth are less likely to be overwhelmed by the intensity of the experience. This may involve reading or attending classes about the birth process or one-on-one instruction from a midwife or childbirth educator. You might observe a friend's birth or watch movies about birth. Learning all you can about the sights, sounds, and sensations you might experience during your own birth can go a long way toward feeling comfortable with the birth process. Most importantly, perhaps, are the breathing, relaxation, massage, self-hypnosis, and meditation skills you'll learn, practice, and develop during your pregnancy. The more you practice, the better prepared you'll be to put these skills to use.

In addition, most women report feeling more comfortable at home than in the hospital, which contributes to feeling more relaxed, which potentially translates to feeling less pain.

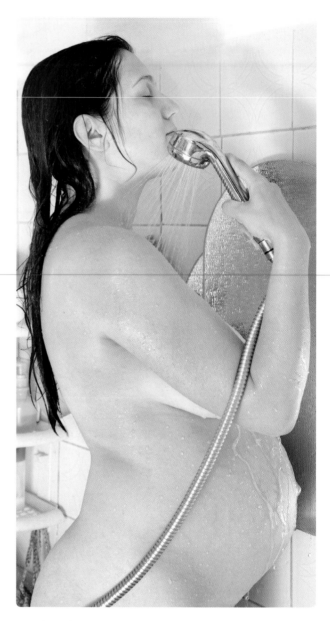

A soothing shower or soaking in warm water can make a big difference in how many women experience pain during labor.

Some women discover, however, that they thought they'd feel good about delivering at home, but when labor actually started, they felt anxious about not being in a health care setting. Their worry about what might happen should an emergency arise overshadowed their comfort level.

If you approach your labor well informed, well supported, and well supplied, the pain you experience during your home birth should be manageable. Here's what you'll need to make your home birth as comfortable as possible:

- A skilled midwife and other health care professionals (acupuncturist, massage therapist, etc.)
- A labor support person or team (your husband or partner, friend, and/or family members, and/or a doula)
- Pain management techniques (like Lamaze breathing and relaxation, HypnoBirthing, meditation, and/or massage skills)
- A bathtub or birthing tub, Jacuzzi, hot tub, shower, or inflatable pool
- Pillows, blankets, and a comfortable bed
- An exercise or yoga ball (a.k.a. birthing ball)
- Other pain management support tools such as tennis balls, a rice sock, and so forth. (see chapter 10)

Is Water Birth Safe?

Some people worry that babies will drown if born underwater, but several naturally occurring physiologic processes prevent that from happening. In addition, the placenta provides oxygen to the baby for a period of time after birth and babies don't usually attempt to take a breath until they reach the water's surface and are exposed to air. In most water births, babies are brought to the water surface and placed upright, skin-to-skin on mom's chest within a few seconds of delivery.

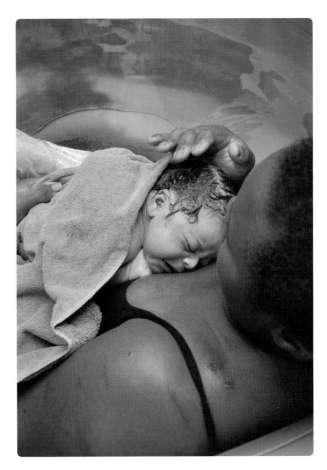

A baby born in water will be brought to the surface and up to mom's chest for skin-to-skin contact within seconds after birth.

Some pediatricians and researchers are concerned about health and safety factors associated with water birth, including the potential for babies to inhale bacteria-contaminated water and contract pneumonia. The American Academy of Pediatrics frowns on water births and in a 2005 statement called them "experimental" because of a lack of studies proving their safety. The academy also says that though there is no evidence that water births cause adverse neonatal or maternal effects, further research is needed to determine their safety.

A Cochrane review of pertinent studies included twelve trials involving 3,243 women and concluded that water births significantly reduced use of epidurals and spinal anesthesia and didn't adversely affect labor, increase need for forceps and vacuum extractors, or adversely affect neonatal well-being. The review, which only relates to water immersion during the first stage of labor, concluded that further research is needed to assess the effect of water births on neonatal and maternal morbidity. No trials were found that assessed the immersion of women in water during the third stage of labor

The bottom line is, there's evidence that laboring and giving birth in water can be great for moms and no solid evidence that directly concludes it is bad for babies. But there's also no evidence to prove it's safe, which pediatricians are concerned about. Some hospitals, however, allow water births at their facilities.

A deep tub full of body-temperature water can help you change positions for pushing and help support you to maintain a squatting position. But some women plan on having a water birth and find they don't actually like it. Don't be so wedded to the

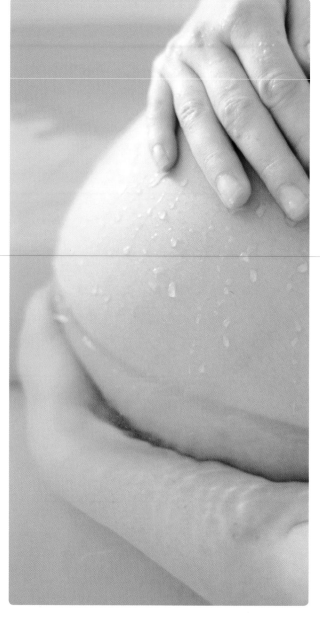

Relaxing in a tub or pool of warm water can relieve anxiety, tension, and pain, and sometimes can even help the progression of labor.

idea of a water birth that you feel disappointed if you end up getting out of the water and giving birth outside the tub.

Water Birth 101

Water birth and home birth can be a perfect combination. Many mothers find laboring in a tub of warm water decreases pain, increases relaxation, and when used with other breathing and relaxation techniques, helps them progress through labor and birth without additional pain management methods.

You can have a water birth in your own tub, but you can also rent or purchase a tub that's specially designed for the job. The tub looks like a deep, inflatable kiddie pool, lined with a disposable plastic liner to ensure it's as clean as possible for each birth. A water birth tub is accessible on all sides, which makes it easier for dad/partner and midwife to support mom and deliver the baby. It's a safe, enclosed space that provides protection.

The tub has to be inflated with a pump and filled with 95°F to 100°F (35°C to 38°C) water. Many women inflate the tub well in advance of labor so it's ready when they need it. Mom can get in the tub whenever she wants or whenever her midwife thinks it's appropriate.

WOULD YOUR DOCTOR OR MIDWIFE DO A HOME BIRTH?

An "attended" home birth is one where a certified nurse midwife, certified midwife, direct entry midwife, or less often, a physician, cares for the laboring woman in her home. An "unattended" home birth is one where the laboring woman is not under the care of a certified professional. She may be giving birth with the help of her partner, a family member, or friend.

Most women who choose to have a home birth work in conjunction with a midwife. About 61 percent of home births from 1990 to 2006 were attended by midwives, including unplanned home births where the baby just came very quickly, according to the CDC. Among those births, 27 percent were delivered by certified nurse midwives and 73 percent were delivered by other midwives. It's worth noting that it is legal in all fifty states to hire a certified nurse midwife, or CNM, to provide care during a home birth, though this practice is rare, as most CNMs work in hospitals. Some certified professional midwives (CPMs) continue to attend mothers in the twenty-three states where it is illegal and can be arrested and prosecuted, while efforts are under way to change the law.

Though no state prosecutes mothers for giving birth outside a hospital, it can be difficult for women to find certified health care practitioners who are willing to attend a home birth. Many feel that it's simply safer to deliver in a health care setting or are prohibited from attending home births by hospital policies and malpractice insurance restrictions.

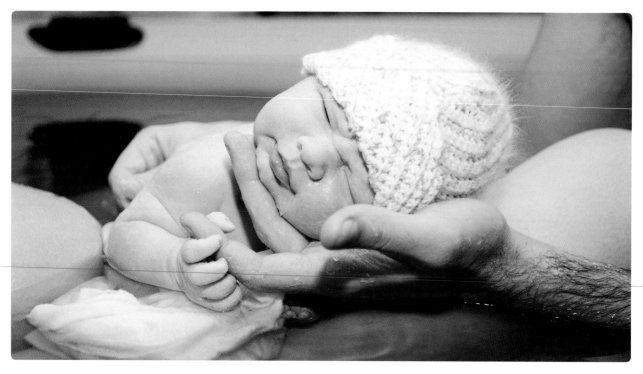

Water-birth babies don't always cry when they're born because warm water and skin-to-skin contact with mom and dad is much like their environment in the uterus.

If you do wish to plan a home birth, seek a certified professional to assist in your care and investigate the laws in the state where you live. It is currently illegal for anyone to practice as a direct entry (i.e., uncertified) midwife attending a home birth in Alabama, Georgia, Hawaii, Illinois, Indiana, Iowa, Kentucky, Maryland, North Carolina, South Dakota, and Wyoming.

Parents who choose to deliver at home deserve to be attended by someone with years of experience, an excellent reputation, a solid education and training background, and a good relationship with a nearby hospital and obstetrician.

It's critical that you do your homework and conduct "background checks" when choosing your home birth provider. Remember, anyone can say she's a midwife, but that doesn't mean she knows what she's doing.

If your midwife is certified and licensed, you have some assurance she's been properly trained and vetted, but many unlicensed direct entry and lay midwives are exceptionally skilled at safe home delivery. Though it's illegal in many states for direct entry midwives to practice, that doesn't necessarily mean midwives in those states don't know what they're doing. It means their state does not have a legal pathway for them to practice. Their ability to practice legally is something you should consider, however, especially if it will affect their ability to transfer care to a hospital in case of emergency.

How Do You Find the Right Midwife?

Word of mouth is a good place to start when searching for the right person to attend your home birth. Ask friends and family members about the midwives they've used, but don't stop there. Check those credentials and references thoroughly.

Here are some excellent online resources for finding a home birth midwife in your area:

- American College of Nurse-Midwives (www.midwife.org/rp/find.cfm). Its database includes CNMs, CMs, CPMs, CNM-NDs, and their contact information or links to their websites.

- Natural Birth Partners (http://birthpartners.com). Its database provides information about all types of midwives as well as doulas, childbirth educators, and other health care providers.

- Midwives Alliance of North America (http://mana.org/). This is a professional organization for midwives from a variety of backgrounds. Referrals can be requested by email.

- American Association of Birth Centers (www.birthcenters.org/find-a-birth-center/). Birth centers and their contact information are listed state by state. Contact birth centers in your area and ask them for referrals to midwives who attend home births.

- North American Registry of Midwives (for certified professional midwives) (http://narm.org/). This professional organization sets the certification standards for CPMs and can provide contact information (via email) for CPMs in your area.

CREATING YOUR EMERGENCY BACKUP PLAN

Though most home births turn out beautifully and result in healthy mothers and babies, serious complications can crop up suddenly during labor or birth. In fact, approximately 15 percent of all pregnancies involve some kind of complication. Though many of those will be spotted during pregnancy (and the patient will be referred to an obstetrician or other specialist for appropriate care), other emergencies spring up unexpectedly during labor. Here are some examples:

- Hemorrhage
- Infection
- High blood pressure and/or preeclampsia
- Eclampsia or seizures of other etiology
- Stroke
- Pulmonary embolism or amniotic fluid embolism
- Prolonged labor or labor that fails to progress
- Umbilical cord accidents (for example, cord gets wrapped around baby or comes down in the vagina in front of the baby's head and cuts off circulation to baby)
- Placental complications (placenta previa—in which the placenta covers the cervix; placenta abruption—in which the placenta separates from the uterine wall before birth)
- Unexpected herpes outbreak, which can result in transfer of herpes to baby and neurologic damage
- Fetal malpresentation (breech, transverse lie)

- Shoulder dystocia (shoulders get trapped in the birth canal)
- Unexpected twin or multiple babies

Different emergency conditions have different symptoms, but here are the most significant ones to watch out for:

- Excessive bleeding
- Foul-smelling amniotic fluid
- High blood pressure
- Rigid abdomen or a contraction that won't relax
- Severe headache
- Weakness or paralysis on one side of the body
- Seeing flashing lights or dots
- Severe upper abdominal pain
- Seizures
- Fainting
- Shortness of breath
- Chest pain or palpitations/feeling of irregular heartbeat
- Thick meconium (baby poop) in the amniotic fluid
- Fever
- Confusion
- Inability to urinate
- Severe vomiting
- Lack of fetal movement
- Delivery of a foot, hand, or other body part before delivery of the head

In addition to these emergencies, there are other conditions (such as maternal exhaustion, inability to handle pain, or unavailability of a midwife) that mean mom should go to the hospital.

Without preparation, many families feel frightened, vulnerable, defensive, and disoriented (in addition to being in pain and exhausted) when they get to the hospital. They may feel like they're out of control. The culture clash between home and hospital can feel harsh.

Hospital staff might feel on guard, too. Patients who come to the hospital for what's called a "failed home birth" are often very sick, and mom, baby, or both might be in serious danger, especially if they've waited too long to transfer care. Mom is usually a stranger to the doctor and hospital who have to start taking care of her "blind" (without the benefit of knowing her). Unless the doctor taking over her care has a relationship with the patient and her midwife, she may not know her medical history. All the doctor knows is she's responsible for an emergency, a mother, and her baby. This is a very stressful situation for everyone involved.

If a woman and her family have prepared for the possibility of transferring, however, it doesn't have to be an alienating crisis. In fact, with the right preparations, it can be a smooth transition for everyone involved. Here's how to prepare for a hospital transfer:

- Don't wait for labor. Start your preparations during your pregnancy.
- Ask your midwife how she manages hospital transfers and under what conditions. She should have a well-established relationship

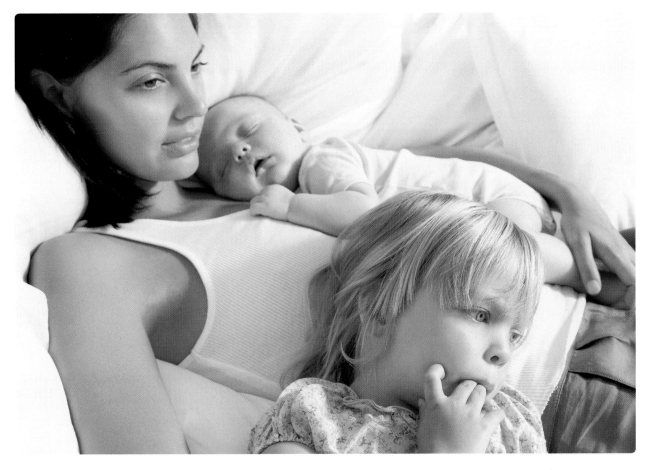

Parents should understand that their birth experience will be vastly different in the hospital than it might be at home. A birthing education program will help families make the right decision for their specific needs.

with an obstetrician who will consult with her and/or assume her patients' care in case of complications or emergencies. If your midwife doesn't have a backup doctor, this is a red flag. Any experienced, qualified midwife should have a solid plan in place (including a backup doctor) to manage emergencies. If she doesn't, find another midwife.

- Make an appointment early in your pregnancy for a meet-and-greet with your midwife's backup doctor. Make sure he or she has a copy of your prenatal records.

- Make an appointment with the doctor late in your pregnancy, so you're familiar with each other.

- Find out what hospital your midwife transfers to and make sure it's the same one where her backup doctor practices and delivers.

- Preregister at the hospital and schedule a tour of its labor and delivery unit. Make sure the hospital has a copy of your prenatal records.

What if you don't like the backup doctor or hospital? Then you have some decisions to make. Chances are good you won't need their services at all. But on the off chance you do, you have to weigh your personal discomfort with that doctor and hospital against your relationship with your midwife. What are your options? You can find another midwife who has a transfer plan you're more comfortable with or find another doctor or hospital willing to take care of you in case of an emergency. There are a lot of liability risks involved with emergency obstetric patients and failed home births. Finding obstetricians willing to take those risks isn't easy.

You can take your chances and just show up at a hospital if an emergency happens in labor. Hospitals are obligated to take care of all emergency patients. Make sure that hospital delivers babies, though. Not all do. Will you get the best possible care? Maybe. Hospital staff will undoubtedly do their best, but if they don't know you at all, they'll be working at a disadvantage.

Some mothers report feeling judged when they come to a hospital after attempting a home birth. Midwives may not want to subject their frightened, overwhelmed patients or themselves to negative scrutiny and judgmental attitudes. Many hospitals recognize that these negative impressions may cause midwives and patients to hesitate (and maybe wait too long) before making the transfer. Considering that more patients are choosing home birth, some hospitals are actively working toward building better standards of care that facilitate smoother transfers with less animosity and conflict.

Patients can do their part by understanding that their birth experience will be different at the hospital than at home (that's why you're transferring, after all), and by familiarizing themselves with the hospital before labor starts. Once you get there, let your doctor do her job. There will be time to discuss, explain, and plan the best course of action to achieve the safest outcome for mom and baby, but your experience will be much more positive if you leave arguments and control issues outside the hospital door. That advice applies to doctors and nurses as well as to patients and their families.

CARE OF MOM AND BABY IMMEDIATELY AFTER A HOME DELIVERY

If you've delivered in bed, then immediately after your baby is born, your midwife will place him on your chest or abdomen for skin-to-skin contact. Her assistant (a nurse, midwife, or other labor support person) will dry baby and make sure he's warm enough, breathing, and becoming pink.

She'll also start observing baby for his Apgar scores. The Apgar score is evaluated at one and five minutes after delivery to determine baby's physical condition and is based on five criteria: heart rate, respiratory effort, muscle tone, response, and skin color. Each criterion is given a value of 0, 1, or 2 points. Scoring a 10 would be considered a perfect score, which very few babies get. An Apgar score that's 8 at one minute and 9 at five minutes would be considered an excellent score.

If you've delivered in a tub, your baby will be brought to the water's surface, placed on your chest, and observed for breathing and Apgar scores. Any assessments your baby needs will be done in your arms. Your midwife might wait for the umbilical cord to stop beating before she clamps it near your baby's tummy. Then, either you, one of your labor support people (baby's dad, your partner, or whomever you've chosen for the honor), or your midwife will cut the cord.

If you've had a water birth, then at this point, it's up to your midwife whether she wants you to move to your bed for the delivery of your placenta. Many midwives feel that the best way for them to evaluate postdelivery bleeding is out of the water and in the bed. Some midwives feel fine evaluating bleeding by just having you stand up or raising your bottom out of the tub.

While your midwife waits for the placenta to be delivered, she'll watch your bleeding carefully and might examine your vagina and perineum for tears or lacerations. While you put baby to breast for the first time or cuddle with your baby, she might start repairing (stitching or suturing) your perineum, deliver your placenta, and continue watching your bleeding. Depending on how well your uterus contracts after the placenta is delivered and how much bleeding is present, she may or may not administer an injection of oxytocin into your thigh or hip or administer misoprostol tablets into your rectum. She or your partner might massage the uterus by vigorously rubbing your lower abdomen to stimulate the uterus to contract and keep postdelivery bleeding to a minimum.

Once she's finished stitching and she's sure you're not bleeding too much, she'll clean you up with warm water and remove wet sheets and pads. She'll place dry padding towels, sheets, and/or large feminine hygiene pads under your bottom and maybe an ice pack to reduce swelling and pain.

After that, you'll be encouraged to rest, breastfeed, and cuddle with your baby. Eventually, your midwife will weigh and measure your baby and do a thorough health assessment on her. You'll be helped up to the bathroom and, if you're not too tired, into the shower. Then you and your baby will be tucked back into bed with snacks, plenty of liquids, and instructions to relax and recover.

The first postpartum day is all about bonding, breastfeeding, bleeding (or making sure you're not bleeding too much), resting, and transitioning into the postpartum period. Your midwife will stay with you for several hours after birth to make sure you and your baby are stable. After that, it'll be up to your partner, family, and/or doula to take care of you. Don't forget about your partner's needs. He's probably been up all night, too, and needs plenty of time for resting, bonding, and recovery.

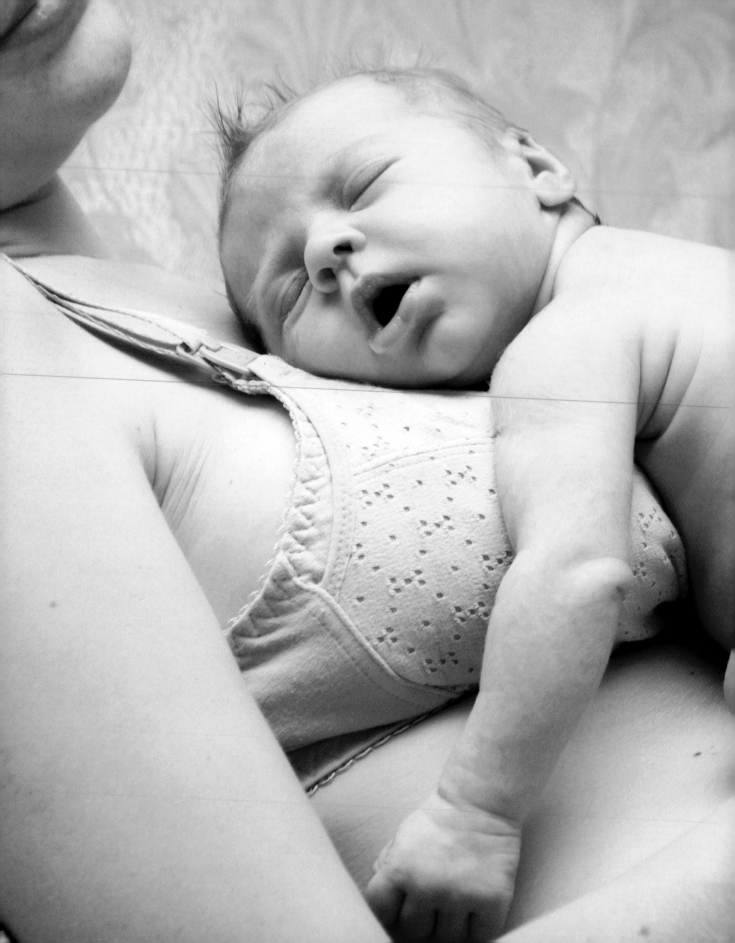

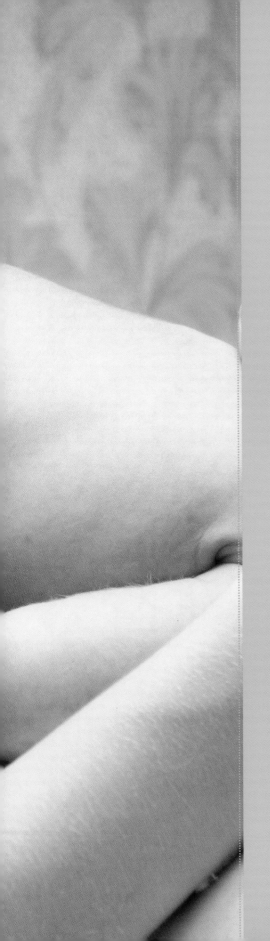

CHAPTER 3

Unmedicated, Vaginal Birth in a Birth Center

What it is, why it may or may not be right for you, pros and cons, and how to prepare for this labor path

For women who expect to have a normal, healthy, low-risk pregnancy and would like to deliver naturally, but who would also like to have access to high-tech help, a birth center may be the perfect option. Birth centers allow you to minimize medical intrusions, while having experts and supplies nearby. If you've got your heart set on a natural delivery, you're more likely to achieve it at a birth center, where natural birth is the norm—you'll have a drug-free birth, rather than use an epidural for labor.

Birth centers generally offer a homelike setting away from your own home. The intimate environment of a birth center might include everything from a living room area for you and your labor team to gather and relax in; a kitchen for you to use throughout your labor; a bedroom with a large bed and linens much like you would have in your own home; and often a large tub for relaxation and water births. Birth centers generally provide more privacy during a delivery, because most birth centers will only have one to three women in labor at any given time, as opposed to the dozens of women you might find in labor at a hospital.

A birth center can be "freestanding," meaning that it's devoted entirely to the care of pregnant and laboring women and is not physically attached to a hospital, or it may be on the grounds of a hospital or within a hospital building or complex.

Birth centers offer complete prenatal care services, diagnostic testing, and labor and delivery facilities and specialists. They're generally staffed by midwives, though you'll also find physicians, nurses, social workers, and parent educators on staff. Most major health insurance plans and Medicaid generally cover birth center care.

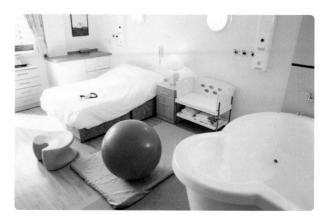

A suite at a birth center is more like home than many standard hospital rooms, but they're also equipped with emergency supplies to facilitate your birth if needed.

HOW A BIRTH CENTER DIFFERS FROM A HOSPITAL

Delivering your baby at a birth center can be very different from what you'd experience in a hospital setting. We've listed the major differences, pros, and cons here.

Pros

- You'll deliver in a comfortable, intimate, home-like environment.
- You can wear your own clothing.
- You can eat and drink whatever you'd like, as your body directs you to.
- You can have a water birth if you choose to do so.

- You can decide whom you'd like to have present at your labor and delivery—including your children, parents, friends, and labor support team.
- You'll have access to labor and delivery specialists and immediate medical care. In the event of an emergency, you can be transferred to a hospital relatively quickly. (According to the American Association of Birth Centers, 12 percent of women in labor typically transfer to a hospital, and the vast majority of these transfers are not emergencies. Only about 2 percent of women transfer for emergency reasons.)
- There are no routine "prep procedures" in a birth center, such as an IV (though your midwife will need to decide whether your individual care dictates needing certain interventions, such as an IV, so you may not be exempt from all procedures).
- Your midwife will stay with you throughout your labor and birth rather than sharing that task with a nurse, as is done in hospitals.

- You can expect to have fewer interventions in a birth center, such as the use of drugs to speed up labor, the use of forceps or vacuum extraction, the use of pain medications, and so on. (A birth center will provide local anesthesia to suture tears in the perineum.)

- There's no continuous electronic fetal monitoring in a birth center, so you won't need to be hooked up to monitors for your entire labor. The reason for this is that patients in a birth center are by definition low risk, and continuous monitoring is not required for these types of patients anywhere, even in a hospital. You will be monitored briefly when you first arrive at the birth center in labor, and your baby's heartbeat will be monitored intermittently with a handheld Doppler device.

- Birth centers are very supportive of natural childbirth and provide many natural techniques for relieving pain, such as the use of birthing balls, massage, movement, warm compresses, Jacuzzis, and so on.

- Birth centers don't routinely perform episiotomies.

- There is no separation of mom and baby in a birth center.

- You can return home shortly after your birth if you wish, or—at some birth centers—transfer to a hospital to stay for up to forty-eight hours after delivery.

- A National Birth Center study reported that 98.8 percent of women using a birth center would recommend it to friends and/or return to the center for a subsequent birth.

- A birth center delivery can cost 30 to 50 percent less than a hospital delivery, according to the American Association of Birth Centers.

Cons

- In many birth centers, the only emergency medical equipment on hand may be oxygen and catheters to clear a baby's airways, if necessary. (If the birth center is connected to a hospital, you'll be transferred to the hospital for additional emergency care.)

- Birth centers typically do not offer anesthesia. Some offer narcotics for pain relief, but not all do. If a mother would like epidural pain relief, she would need to be transferred to the hospital.

- In the event of complications, it would be necessary to transfer to a hospital. (If you choose a freestanding birth center and you need to be transferred to a hospital, there may be a delay in lifesaving care for you and your baby.)

- Birth centers are not readily available in many parts of the United States.

- You'll typically need to leave the birth center within six to twelve hours after giving birth (though you can usually transfer to an affiliated hospital to stay for up to forty-eight hours after giving birth).

Inside Information

Insurance providers are part of every birth plan at every hospital and most birth centers. Though doctors, midwives, nurses, and hospitals are committed to providing the best obstetric care possible, it's a fact of modern medicine that insurance providers heavily influence the way they take care of their patients. That's because labor and delivery is a high litigation target area.

If something happens to mom or baby and the family sues the doctor, midwife, labor nurse, or hospital (or all four), the insurance company payout can be very high—that is, if the patient wins a financial settlement. Patients don't usually win these cases, but lengthy court cases still affect the price of obstetric care. That means obstetricians and midwives pay some of the highest malpractice insurance premiums of all medical specialties. Hospitals draft strict guidelines and standards of care to keep their patients healthy and their doctors and staff out of the courtroom.

These reasons are partly why hospital-based labor and delivery units tend to use more medical interventions than birth centers (many patients in the hospital actually need more interventions) and why only healthy pregnant women with minimal risks for complications are allowed to deliver in a birth center. Women with increased risk factors are generally not allowed to use a birth center for their delivery.

Patients' risk factors are assessed throughout pregnancy to make sure a birth center delivery remains appropriate. Sometimes a woman who is healthy and eligible for a birth center delivery at the beginning of her prenatal care will develop risk factors during the pregnancy. Maybe her weight climbs too high or she has elevated blood pressure at one of her prenatal appointments. If she develops complications—such as insulin-dependent diabetes or preeclampsia—she may "risk out."

Having increased risk factors doesn't necessarily mean her health conditions will interfere with her ability to have a natural or vaginal birth. They also don't mean she's likely to have prenatal complications or problems during labor. In fact, she's still far more likely to have an entirely normal and healthy pregnancy and birth than she is to develop complications. On paper, however, her midwife might not be able to afford taking any chances by having her deliver at a birth center.

Some patients go through their entire pregnancy only to "risk out" at the end. Maybe they go past their due date or their baby measures larger than normal. Sometimes midwives will still lean toward a birth center delivery, but with the understanding that they might transfer care if there's any complication. Does that mean that mother can't deliver naturally, vaginally, and with her midwife caring for her? Not at all. She can still have a natural birth, but her midwife might have to follow the regulations mandated by the hospital instead of the more relaxed standards of a birth center.

Different birth centers have different criteria for eligibility. Ask your midwife or doctor about his or her criteria for being risked out and how your health conditions could affect your ability to deliver at a birth center.

WHO CAN—AND CAN'T—DELIVER AT A BIRTH CENTER?

Birth centers are intended for women who expect to have a healthy, low-risk pregnancy.

You may not be able to deliver at a birth center if:

- You're pregnant with multiples. Some birth centers will deliver twins, but you have to ask.

- You have a chronic health condition such as diabetes, high blood pressure, or a seizure or other disorder.

- You've had a previous Cesarean delivery. Some birth centers will do a vaginal birth after C-section, but you need to ask.

- You are obese.

- You use tobacco or illegal drugs.

Why You May Be "Risked Out" of a Birth Center

Keep in mind that even if you are having a normal, healthy pregnancy, you may be "risked out" of a birth center birth at any point during your pregnancy or labor if you develop any of the following complications or other risk factors that your midwife feels necessitate transfer out of birth center care:

- Preeclampsia

- High blood pressure

- Severe anemia

- Polyhydramnios (elevated levels of amniotic fluid) or oligohydramnios (not enough amniotic fluid)

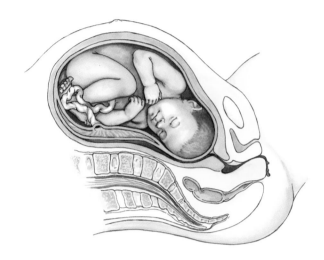

Placental abruption. A normal placenta is attached along the side of the uterus and nowhere near the cervix. Here, the placenta has detached from the uterus, which dramatically reduces maternal-fetal circulation and may result in hemorrhage.

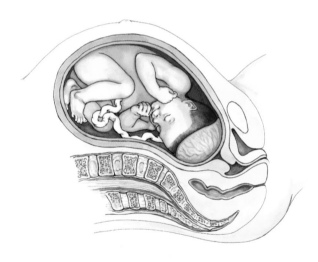

Placenta previa. The placenta lies across the opening to the cervix in front of the baby's head. There is no way to have a safe vaginal birth with placenta previa.

- Placenta previa (where the placenta covers all or part of the opening to the cervix)
- Placental abruption (where the placenta is pulling away from the uterine wall)
- A breech or malpositioned baby
- Preterm or late-term delivery (before 37 weeks or after 42 weeks)
- Your baby has a known medical problem (such as a heart defect)

HOW TO FIND A BIRTH CENTER—AND HOW TO CHECK OUT ITS REPUTATION

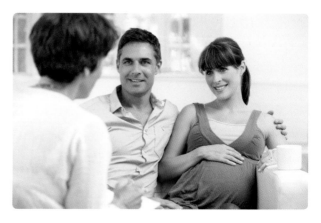

Birth centers can vary in their philosophies and styles. Do your homework, ask lots of questions, and check references. Take a tour before deciding whether it's where you want to have your baby.

Birth centers can vary in their philosophies and practices, so it's important to do your research. The first thing you'll want to find out is whether the birth center is nationally accredited by the Commission for the Accreditation of Birth Centers, and licensed in your state. Start your search for accredited birth centers by state at the American Association of Birth Centers website, at www.birthcenters.org/find-a-birth-center. You'll also want to call your insurance provider to ask about coverage details for birth center care.

Once you've found a birth center in your area, schedule a visit to tour the facility, meet the staff, and ask yourself the following questions:

- Is the birth center within a reasonable driving distance from your home? You'll need to be there frequently for prenatal visits and you won't want to have a long drive when you're in labor. If you live far from the birth center, decide whether the distance is manageable.

- Does the birth center seem clean and well organized?
- Do you like the birth center environment in general? Do you feel comfortable there?
- Does the birth center staff seem professional and personable?

You'll want to ask the birth center staff the following questions:

- Are the staff members who will attend my labor and delivery licensed health care providers (e.g., physicians, nurse-midwives, or licensed midwives)? What are their credentials?
- Is the birth center affiliated with a hospital? If so, which one?
- Who is the consulting physician for the birth center?
- Do the birth center health care providers have hospital privileges? (If not, are they able to stay with me throughout the delivery in the event of a hospital transfer?)

- How does the birth center handle complications during pregnancy, labor, and delivery?

- What do I do if I have a medical question or emergency after hours?

- In what situations, if any, would the birth center induce labor with Pitocin (oxytocin) or by breaking the amniotic sac (amniotomy)?

- Does the birth center offer any analgesic drugs?

- What if I decide that I'd like to have an epidural during labor?

- What sort of electronic fetal monitoring does the center do?

- Are there any time limits placed on labor?

- How does the birth center handle transfers to a hospital?

- How long does it take to transfer mom and baby to the hospital?

- What types of insurance does the birth center accept? (Does the birth center accept my insurance?)

- Can I have a water birth?

- How will the staff assist me during labor?

- What are the birth center's statistics on episiotomies, assisted deliveries with forceps or suction, hospital transfers, and so forth? A hospital transfer rate of 7 to 12 percent is reasonable and an episiotomy rate of less than 10 percent is considered acceptable, according to the American Pregnancy Association. Vacuum deliveries comprised 4.1 percent of all live births in 2004, and 1.1 percent of babies were delivered via forceps. Your birth center's assisted delivery statistics should be well below these rates.

Even in this information age, it can't hurt to ask for word-of-mouth testimonials from women who've used a birth center. Ask friends and family—or Google the facility to see what you find online.

The Dearth of Birth Centers

When you begin your search for a birth center, you may be surprised to find that there just aren't that many! For the past few years, birth centers around the country have been closing their doors. Some of the reasons cited for all the closures have been the rising cost of malpractice insurance premiums, lagging insurance company reimbursements, and a lack of physicians and hospitals willing to provide backup care because of an increasing fear of lawsuits.

In addition, birth centers have found themselves in competition with hospitals that are now offering a more homelike environment. Though these same pressures are being felt in hospitals around the country, birth centers are particularly vulnerable because their low-intervention, low-cost procedures aren't offset by the higher revenues that hospitals see from higher-paying procedures. Many of the birth centers that are surviving have been forced to rely on private donations and grants to keep their doors open.

About Fetal Monitoring

Three types of monitoring devices are used in various types of birth settings: handheld, external, and internal monitoring:

- Handheld devices are used for intermittent monitoring and include Dopplers (a small ultrasound device) and fetoscopes (looks and operates like a stethoscope with a bell-shaped piece that's applied to mom's stomach) to amplify baby's heartbeat. Handheld devices are used at home, birth centers, and hospitals.

- An external fetal monitor is a disc-shaped ultrasound device that's placed on mom's stomach with a belt or Velcro strap. The baby's heartbeat is amplified and simultaneously recorded on a computer and paper strip. It can be used for intermittent or continuous monitoring in birth centers, providers' offices, and hospitals.

- An internal fetal monitor is threaded through mom's vagina and attached by a tiny wire directly to baby's scalp. It provides direct measurement of baby's heartbeat (rather than measuring it indirectly through mom's abdomen) by EKG and is considered the most accurate way to evaluate baby's heartbeat. It is only used for continuous monitoring when mom's amniotic membrane is ruptured and in special circumstances where external monitoring is inadequate and usually only in hospital birth settings.

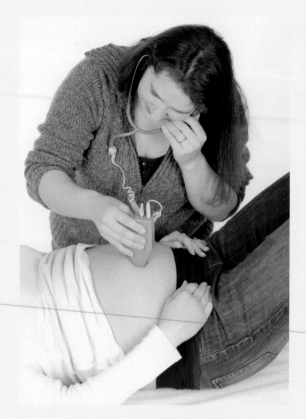

Handheld devices such as this Doppler are used to amplify baby's heartbeat in providers' offices, at home, in birth centers, and during hospital births. Your baby's heartbeat gives clues as to how she's tolerating pregnancy and birth.

CREATE AN EMERGENCY BACKUP PLAN IF YOU GET TRANSFERRED TO A HOSPITAL

Research has generally shown that for healthy, low-risk pregnancies, outcomes for mom and babies are the same in birth centers as they are in hospitals. In fact, many studies argue that—for normal, low-risk pregnancies—delivering in a birth center can be safer for mom and baby than delivering in a hospital because of a decrease in interventions that can lead to complications.

Most birth center labors and deliveries are uncomplicated and safe, but once in a while, emergencies happen. That means you'll need an emergency backup plan to transfer to a hospital with a labor and delivery unit and maybe a NICU.

If you're delivering in a birth center that's connected to a hospital, your midwife will place you in a wheelchair or onto a gurney and push you over to the hospital. She might continue comanaging your care with a physician or she might turn your care over to a doctor. If your birth center is located some

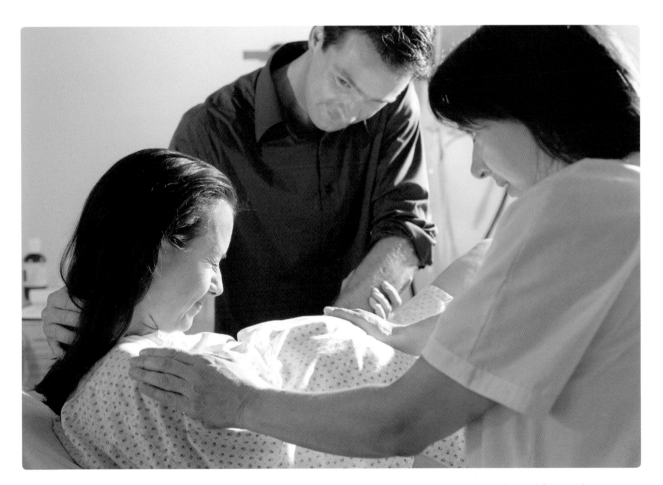

For healthy, low-risk pregnancies, outcomes for moms and babies are the same or better in birth centers as they are in hospitals because they use fewer interventions.

distance away, you'll need transportation. Depending on how big the emergency is, you'll either go by ambulance or in your own car. Make sure your driver knows where the hospital is.

One of the benefits of using birth centers staffed by certified nurse-midwives and connected (either by location or by their professional association) to a hospital is that they already have a system in place for transfers and emergencies. There's an obstetrician assigned to care for emergency patients, and your prenatal records are probably already on-site. The obstetrician probably knows your midwife and understands the midwife model of care. CNMs at hospital-based birth centers tend to err on the side of caution more than some other types of midwives. That means they might transfer care sooner or under less ominous emergency circumstances than some other midwives might. It also means their patients might be better prepared for the hospital experience.

The relationship between your midwife and the admitting OB is important. If they know and respect each other, that attitude will transfer to their patient's experience. If they distrust each other or there's animosity between them, the patient may end up feeling like she's not getting the respect she deserves. This may be less of an issue when the birth center has a direct relationship with the hospital. The hospital staff will already know the midwife, so there very likely will be less tension than for a lay midwife who has no affiliation with the hospital.

If you're using a birth center that's not already connected to a hospital, you'll want to make sure

well in advance of labor that an emergency system is in place. The best way to do that is by making an appointment during your pregnancy to meet the doctor assigned for backup emergencies, become familiar with the hospital, tour the labor and delivery unit, and make sure the hospital has your prenatal records. That way, you won't be a stranger to the staff there.

Once you're at the hospital, you'll be admitted to a labor room for evaluation. Expect a doctor to come in and introduce herself to you as a new member of your health care team. You should also expect continuous fetal heart monitoring (at least for a while) and maybe a vaginal exam. You might receive an IV and lab tests. If you've transferred for a non-life-threatening reason (for example, you want an epidural or your labor has stalled), you might stay in your labor room until you deliver. Your husband/partner and/or midwife can stay with you. The rest of your family might be allowed to stay, but that depends on hospital visiting policies.

If your emergency is a biggie (which means you or your baby are in potential danger), you might be whisked to the operating room. You'll get an IV and lab work quickly. In addition to your obstetrician, you might also meet her partners, an anesthetist (or anesthesiologist), possibly a pediatrician, and a team of nurses and support staff.

Your doctors (and hopefully your midwife, too) will give you a brief explanation of what your emergency is and what they plan to do about it (for example, an immediate C-section). There may not be time for a lengthy discussion at this time. But when the delivery is over and everyone is safe, you and your doctors will have a more complete conversation and they'll answer all your questions.

If you need a C-section, things will move very quickly. If there's time for spinal anesthesia, your husband/partner will most likely be able to stay with you. If there's no time, and you need general anesthesia (which means you go to sleep), your support people will not be allowed in the operating room. That's nonnegotiable in virtually all hospitals, because general anesthesia requires doctors to work at a faster pace and with minimal distractions (e.g., anxious fathers).

After-delivery care depends on whether you delivered vaginally or by C-section and whether you had an epidural, spinal, or general anesthesia. Immediate care for baby depends on his condition after birth.

What's ACOG's Position on Birth Centers?

In 2011, the American Congress of Obstetricians and Gynecologists (ACOG) issued a statement on "out-of-hospital births" that opens with "Although the Committee on Obstetric Practice believes that hospitals and birthing centers are the safest setting for birth, it respects the right of a woman to make a medically informed decision about delivery."

ACOG defines a birth center as an accredited and properly credentialed entity that functions as an extension of the hospital system. In other words, ACOG thinks *birth center* and *hospital* are basically the same type of medical place offering the same type of medical care, as long as there are proper credentials and licensed practitioners available, and consultation with hospital staff is done in a timely and appropriate manner. ACOG's 2011 statement reflects its long-held belief that a hospital—or a birth center within a hospital complex—is the safest place to give birth. It does not officially support giving birth in other settings (such as a birth center that's unaffiliated with a hospital).

In response to ACOG's position on home birth, in 2006, the American College of Nurse-Midwives (ACNM), in conjunction with the American Association of Birth Centers, the American Nurses Association, Birth Network National, Citizens for Midwifery, the Coalition for Improving Maternity Services, Lamaze International, Midwives Alliance of North America, and the White Ribbon Alliance for Safe Motherhood, said the following:

"We are not aware of evidence supporting the assertion that the hospital is the safest setting for labor, birth and the immediate postpartum period for low risk women . . . We encourage ACOG to partner with other health care providers to enhance the safety of birth in out-of-hospital settings by promoting an agenda for continued research, developing policies to ensure seamless coordination of care across settings, and encouraging collaborative management across disciplines. ACNM proposes the development of a joint task force to develop guidelines for out-of-hospital birth and to establish a research agenda to explore issues of safety across birth settings."

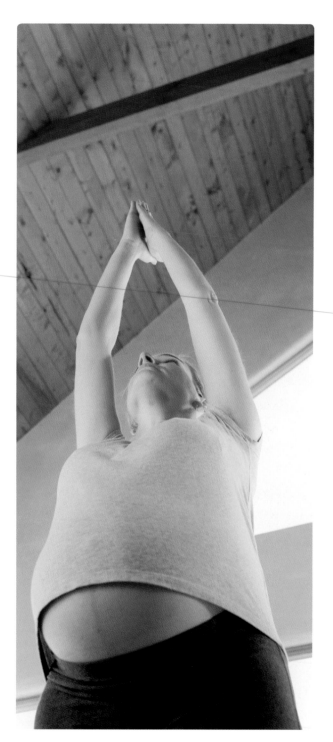

One of the best ways to ensure you won't risk out for a birth center birth is to support your health throughout your pregnancy.

How to Prepare for a Birth Center Delivery

To get ready for a birth center delivery, you'll want to focus on childbirth education programs, books, and information that support natural delivery and that view labor and delivery as a "normal" event in a woman's life—not one that necessitates medical care in a hospital. Choose childbirth education programs that have a holistic view of pregnancy and labor, such as HypnoBirthing, the Bradley Method, Lamaze, or Birthing From Within. Your birth center may have a lending library that offers books and other information that support its personal philosophy of giving birth.

When it comes time to pack your bag for a birth center delivery, you'll be delighted to find that in addition to the regular items you'll find on a "What to Pack for the Hospital" list, you'll also be able to pack food to sustain you and your labor team during labor and delivery. Your birth center may even allow you to bring a celebratory bottle of champagne—provided that you limit yourself to one glass!

What Happens after the Delivery?

If you deliver in a birth center, your baby will be placed in your arms immediately, and you'll be allowed to keep your baby with you at all times thereafter. Your midwife may suction the baby's mouth and nose to clear the airway of any fluids then or as the baby's head emerges from the birth canal. She'll typically clamp the umbilical cord in two places after it stops pulsing and will often have your labor partner cut the cord. (Your midwife may

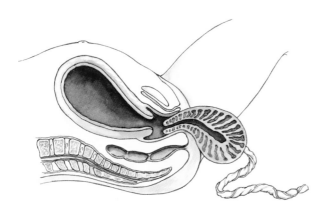

Delivery of a normal, healthy placenta *usually happens within thirty minutes after birth and is relatively painless. Since it is made up of only soft tissues, it slips out of the vagina easily.*

collect blood from the umbilical cord to check your baby's blood type and for other possible tests.)

Your midwife will examine the baby while she lies on your chest, deliver the placenta, and repair any tearing in your perineum. She'll examine you to ensure that you're not experiencing excessive bleeding or other complications (she may massage your uterus to encourage it to begin contracting). She'll check vital signs for you and your baby, including temperature, pulse, and heart rate. At one and five minutes after birth, an Apgar assessment will be done to evaluate baby's heart rate, breathing, muscle tone, reflex response, and color. Your midwife will encourage you to try breastfeeding as soon as possible.

Within an hour after delivery, your baby will be weighed at your bedside, and your midwife will also footprint your baby. Your baby might receive some immediate care such as antibiotic eye ointment to prevent infection (required by law in many states) and a vitamin K injection to help baby's blood clot.

(Some women decline various medications for themselves or their babies. In this instance, your midwife would review the issues with you and have you sign a form saying that you've declined treatment.)

Assuming that you and your baby are healthy and doing well, most birth centers will allow a new family to remain in the birth room for six to twelve hours. At that point, you can either go straight home or transfer to the hospital's maternity floor, where the nursing staff will help care for you and your baby for up to forty-eight hours after delivery. If you do choose to go home, it is important that you get up to use the bathroom without getting dizzy; that your baby nurses well; and that you have a good meal and a well-deserved nap. Your pediatrician may want to see the baby for an office visit within the first twenty-four hours after delivery.

Follow-up care may include a phone call from your midwife, a home visit, lactation support, and/or an office visit within two weeks of your delivery. Assuming that you and your baby are recovering well from labor and delivery and adjusting to your new life together at home, you won't need to see your midwife again until you have a postpartum checkup at six weeks after delivery. In the meantime, you can expect that your baby will see her pediatrician for a one-week, two-week, four-week, and six-week checkup, and you should always call your midwife or birth center if you have any questions, challenges, or complications along the way.

Understanding Mandatory Care

Let's say you want a "birth center–style" natural delivery at the hospital, and you want it to be as close as possible to a home birth. You want to avoid excess fetal monitoring, labor and deliver in a tub, and be able to eat, drink, and move around however and whenever you want. This might be the way to go for women who don't live near a birth center or whose families/partners aren't comfortable with an out-of-hospital birth.

But when you get to the labor unit, your nurse hands you a hospital gown and tells you to change and get into bed. She attaches you to the fetal heart monitor, puts on a blood pressure cuff (set to check your blood pressure automatically every fifteen minutes), starts asking you questions, and enters your information into the computer. Then she says she's going to draw your blood for labor work and start an IV. Oh, and she's going to do a vaginal exam, too. Then she leaves you alone, hooked up to equipment. You begin to wonder where your natural birth plans went.

How much of the nurse's care plan is mandatory and how much is just routine? How much can you opt out of? If you're entirely healthy, have no increased risk factors, and your pregnancy has been smooth the whole way through, you can opt out of quite a lot. You can wear your own clothes, get up and walk, labor in the tub, and have a natural and homelike delivery. Your nurse does, however, have to establish that you and your baby have a healthy baseline and remain at low risk during your labor. This requires a certain amount of medical care, including the following:

- **Computer documentation:** Paper charting is obsolete in almost every hospital nowadays. Your nurse's job is to document every step of your labor, and that means increasing amounts of computer charting. This isn't optional.

- **Fetal heart monitoring:** You have to be on the monitor for at least twenty minutes, possibly longer, at the beginning of your labor and then at regular intervals (called intermittent monitoring) until you deliver. When your nurse has a "good-looking" monitor strip, she can take the belts off. If she needs more time because she doesn't have the right information yet, try to be patient.

Your nurse is looking for what's known as a Category 1 tracing. That means baby's heart is at a normal baseline (usually between 110 and 160 beats per minute) with no decelerations (it doesn't slow down in one of several ominous-looking patterns that sometimes indicate problems). It also has to demonstrate "variability," which means that the heart rate fluctuates between six and twenty-five beats around the baseline (a sign of well-being). She also wants to see accelerations (baby's heart rate increases by fifteen beats or more for at least fifteen seconds). If baby does all that in the first twenty minutes—excellent. If your baby's taking a nap during your monitoring session, however, and the strip doesn't meet criteria to be Category 1, then your nurse can't document that. There's probably nothing wrong with your baby and, in fact, fetal heart monitoring is notoriously inaccurate at predicting babies who really are in trouble. Still, fetal heart monitoring is the standard that hospital (and birth center) obstetric care is based on. It's a huge part of your nurse's job and she has to do it.

A note about fetal heart monitor evaluations:

- Category 1 means baby looks normal and there's nothing to worry about.
- Category 2 means something looks questionable and requires interventions, but it's not necessarily alarming.
- Category 3 is ominous. Sound the alarms and do something! Either get that baby out now (vaginally or by C-section) or do some other intervention to improve the situation.

- **Vital signs:** Your nurse has to check your blood pressure, pulse, respirations, reflexes, and temperature as part of her basic assessment and occasionally throughout your care. Once she has her numbers, though, she can take that equipment off and you don't have to remain hooked up to anything.

- **IV and lab work:** These items are usually optional. Because most hospital patients get IVs and blood tests, it might be part of your nurse's routine to tick this off her to-do list shortly after your admission. It's a whole lot easier to start an IV and draw lab work when the patient is not in hard-rockin' labor, begging for an epidural, or being wheeled to the operating room. Your nurse might also be pressured by her supervisors to have her patients ready for anything that might happen during labor, including surgery.

  If you don't want an IV and your nurse doesn't have a compelling reason why you need one, just say no. If she tells you it's mandatory, ask her why, who says so, and that you want to discuss it with your midwife or doctor. If you're healthy, don't want or need pain medication or any other drugs during labor, and you can drink fluids and keep them down, you don't necessarily need an IV. If you develop complications that require an IV or blood to be drawn, your nurse, a lab technician, or IV specialist can manage that quickly later.

Try not to argue or be too defensive if you and your nurse don't see eye to eye. Not every nurse is comfortable taking care of patients who want to use natural or birth center techniques. For that nurse, it's a little like going without a safety net. Tell her how you envision your labor going, what interventions you want to avoid, and ask for her support. If she can't be supportive or you feel like she's pressuring you, discuss your concerns with your doctor or midwife (who presumably knows your birth plans and preferences and has more authority than your nurse does) and ask for a different nurse.

Be flexible and don't assume that all interventions are unnecessary. Complications happen quickly in labor and delivery, and your nurse has a lot of experience. Many of those problems can be solved quickly with minor interventions.

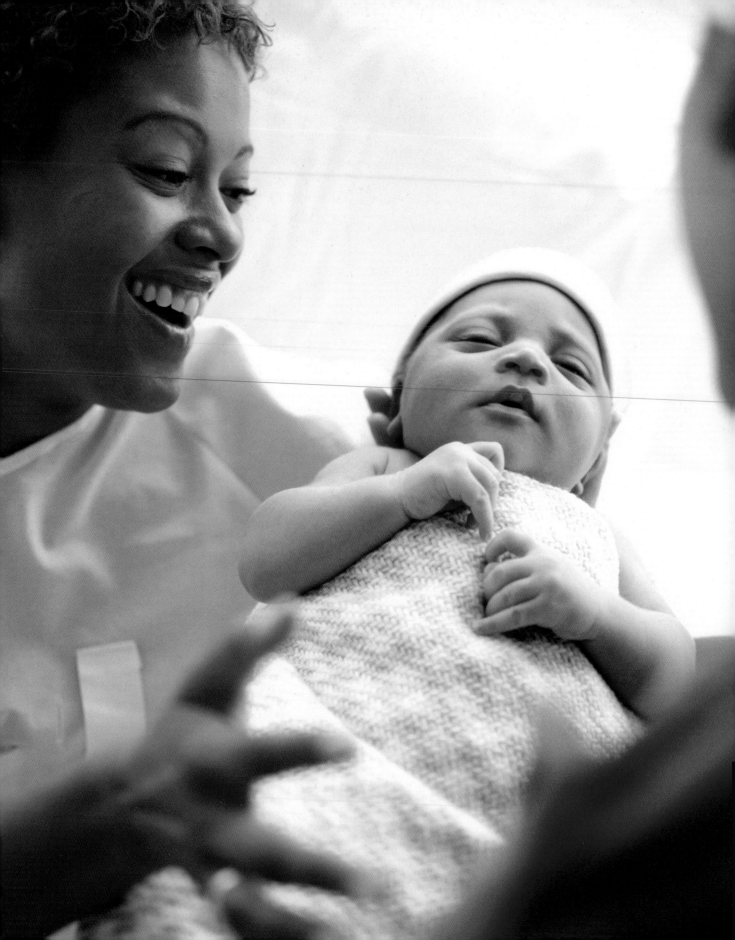

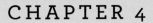
Unmedicated, Vaginal Birth in a Hospital

What it is, why it may or may not be right for you, pros and cons, and how to prepare for this labor path

Many women approach labor wanting a natural birth, but they know an out-of-hospital delivery isn't for them. Maybe their insurance provider won't pay for a home birth or there's no birth center in their area. Maybe they don't feel entirely safe about delivering outside a hospital or they have a medical condition that bears watching. Maybe a woman wants an out-of-hospital birth, but her family doesn't feel comfortable with it, so she bows to their wishes. For as many reasons as there are to plan a natural birth, there are just as many reasons to plan to have it in a hospital.

As of the latest statistics, 98.9 percent of American women deliver in the hospital and a high percentage of those (especially first-time mothers) go into labor intending to have a natural birth. But hospitals aren't always the most conducive locations for using natural childbirth techniques. Consider these statistics:

- About 71 percent of mothers wind up having epidurals for pain relief.
- Ninety percent of mothers have continuous fetal heart monitoring.
- Eighty percent have IVs.
- Only 24 percent walk around during labor after being admitted to the hospital.
- Only 68 percent have vaginal deliveries.
- About 5 percent of vaginal births involve the use of either forceps or vacuum extraction.

WHY DO SO FEW NATURAL BIRTHS OCCUR IN HOSPITALS?

There are many reasons. When a woman delivers at home or in a birth center, there's an implicit understanding that she'll have a natural birth. She is healthy and at low risk for complications. Plus, there simply isn't any option for pain relief other than "going natural."

Hospitals, on the other hand, are loaded with pain relief options and are the experts at providing it. More patients come to deliver at a hospital wanting pain management than not. In addition, many first-time mothers who intend to "go natural" have no real idea what labor is like when they're in

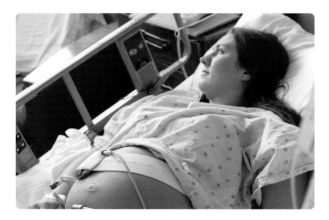

Even with extra procedures like fetal heart monitoring, having a natural birth in the hospital is entirely possible. In fact, for some women, it provides the best chance for having a safe, vaginal birth.

the planning stage and once they find out, wind up changing their birth plans.

Hospitals take care of a broad range of patients. Some are healthy and some aren't. Some need medical interventions and some don't. Some want a natural birth and some don't. Doctors and midwives often practice a different model of care in the hospital than midwives do in out-of-hospital facilities. Plus, insurance and hospital policies dictate certain standards of care and interventions that are considered routine for most patients. If a patient doesn't want those interventions, she has to actively opt out.

That being said, having a natural birth in the hospital is entirely possible and is the best place for many women to deliver, especially if they have increased risks for complications. Achieving a natural birth in the hospital takes planning, education, and the right support (including the right physician, midwife, and labor nurse, a primary labor support person, and maybe a doula). It also takes some finesse at discussing and negotiating certain routine hospital procedures, the willingness to try a variety of labor techniques, and a trusting relationship with your health care providers.

Pros and Cons of Having an Unmedicated Birth in the Hospital

There are lots of plusses for having an unmedicated delivery in the hospital, but there are also some minuses. Here are the pros and cons of having a natural birth in the hospital:

Pros

- Hospitals have everything you need for labor and delivery including supplies, expert personnel, and a private space.

- Your insurance covers hospital birth (and might not cover a home or birth center birth).

- You don't have to transfer care from home or a birth center to the hospital if there's an emergency.

- Some hospitals have cozy, homelike private rooms with sleeping and kitchen accommodations for families.

- Natural birth techniques/processes might be strongly encouraged and supported, including water birth in some hospitals.

- Most hospitals encourage breastfeeding and rooming in and have the nurses, lactation specialists, and other staff available to support you.

- Nurses are available around the clock to support your personal-care needs; assist in your labor, delivery, and recovery process; and keep a close eye on you and your baby during the immediate postpartum period.

- You can request a nurse who enjoys working with "natural birth" patients.

- The nursery is available to provide respite care for you and special care for your newborn if she needs help transitioning to her new life.

- Your hospital might use hospitalists (also known as laborists)—doctors who stay in the labor unit and specialize in supervising labor and delivery patients. You probably won't have met the hospitalist prior to delivery, but hospitals are using these doctors to reduce doctor fatigue and medical errors, increase availability of VBACs, and potentially lower C-section rates.

- You don't have to do your own (or your family's) laundry, housekeeping, or meal preparation for a couple of days after birth.

- Hospital staff can be your "privacy gatekeepers" by helping you reduce or limit visitors if you're overwhelmed, or if you have visitors who are negatively influencing your birth experience.

Cons

- Pain management options and medical interventions are readily available, which makes it easier to slide into a medicated birth. Nurses and doctors focus on hospital standards of care and have direct access to and support for using medical interventions. They may be more likely to use them if they're readily available.

- You may be allowed to use a bathtub and/or Jacuzzi for labor, but only if someone else isn't already using it.

- Most hospitals don't allow delivery in the tub.

- You won't get to handpick your labor nurse and can't guarantee you'll get one who's a good match for your birthing philosophy.

- The doctor or midwife you saw during your pregnancy might not be the one on call when you're in labor.

- If your labor progresses slowly, you might be encouraged to augment the pace with medical interventions, like rupture of the membranes (that's when the midwife or doctor breaks the amniotic sac or water bag with a plastic hook) and Pitocin.

- There may be less one-on-one support than you'd receive at home and less flexibility for how, where, and when you can move around and deliver.

- Hospital staff tend to see patients differently than home and birth center midwives do. Though the Midwives' Model of Care sees birth as an essentially normal, healthy process, hospital staff sees it as potentially risky. This shift in perspective influences many health care providers' care practices.

- Pressure to go with the hospital flow rather than to opt out of interventions can be intimidating.

- Hospitals aren't as quiet, mellow, and private as your home is. There may be dozens of women in labor at the same time.

- Hospitals expose you and your family to germs you wouldn't encounter at home (though all staff are trained in aseptic techniques).

- A lot of people you don't know from many different departments will be part of your hospital care, from admissions personnel to lab technicians, nurses, doctors, and more.

- You may or may not have a private room and bathroom.

- You may or may not be allowed to shower or bathe when you want.

- You may or may not be allowed to eat and drink whenever you want.

- You might not get as much uninterrupted rest as you need because staff will come in and out of your room frequently.

- Even if you choose "rooming in," your baby might be taken to the nursery for routine tests.

- Babies receive more blood tests and medical interventions in hospitals.

- If your labor suite isn't also a postpartum room, you might have to move rooms shortly after your delivery.

- There may be limits on how many visitors you can have and when they can visit you.

HOW TO PREPARE FOR A NATURAL BIRTH IN THE HOSPITAL

There's a lot to plan for and consider when you're working toward a natural birth.

How do you choose a provider (OB, midwife, family practice physician, labor and delivery nurse) who supports low-intervention births? Choosing the right provider for your prenatal care is among the most important decisions you'll make toward achieving your natural birth. If that provider has a reputation for using as few interventions as possible and supporting natural techniques and a lower than average C-section rate, then he or she might be a good match.

Midwives tend to be "more natural" than doctors (they take care of the least risky patients) and family practice doctors "more natural" than OBs, because the OBs are the ones taking care of the higher-risk patients. Don't let their job title be your biggest deciding factor. We've all worked with midwives who were high interventionists and OBs who practice a lot like midwives.

Ask your friends and family for their recommendations. Call the hospital and ask which providers are most supportive of natural births and have the lowest C-section rates. Contact the American College of Nurse Midwives and find out about hospital-based midwives in your area. When in labor, ask to be assigned to a nurse who is supportive and experienced at taking care of natural birth patients.

The choices you make during pregnancy pave the way to the type of delivery you might have. If you want a low-intervention birth, try to opt for a low-intervention pregnancy. Stay healthy to avoid the need for extra health testing and interventions. Ask your provider which screening and diagnostic tests are mandatory and which are optional. Educate yourself about standard, routine, and special tests so you're prepared to make active decisions with your provider about which ones are appropriate for you.

How to prepare to manage your pain without drugs. With the possible exception of a birthing tub, you can use all the same pain management techniques discussed in chapters 2 and 3 in the hospital. Many hospitals have traditional bathtubs, Jacuzzis, and even birthing tubs. Lamaze, Hypno-Birthing, the Bradley Method, and Birthing From Within all offer techniques that can work in any setting. Massage, position changes, birthing balls, walking, showers—any of these strategies can work well in a hospital.

We'll discuss natural pain management techniques further in chapter 10. The key to dealing with pain during labor is to ask your support people to encourage and support the natural techniques you've prepared and to recommend other methods that might help. Ask them to keep offers and recommendations for pain medication or an epidural on the sidelines or don't offer them at all. We'll talk about this further in this chapter's Real Deal.

Hospitals that care for a lot of high-risk patients will have higher C-section and epidural rates and might use more interventions than hospitals that take care of primarily low-risk patients, but they can accommodate low-risk, natural patients, too. In the end, a hospital's reputation and how you feel when you tour it are your best deciding factors.

Inside Information

Many women (especially first-time mothers) come to the hospital prepared to fight for their right to deliver naturally. It doesn't always have to be a fight, however, especially if you've chosen a doctor or midwife with a solid reputation for supporting unmedicated, low-intervention birth, a low C-section rate, and a good relationship with hospital staff.

Contrary to the bad PR we get, many doctors, nurses, and hospital staff members actually like natural births. They're invigorating and renew our faith in a woman's ability to work with her own body and our commitment to help women have their best births possible. That's our goal—the best birth possible—whether we're hospital-, birth center-, or home-based.

When you're ready to leave for the hospital, call ahead and ask for a labor nurse who enjoys working with "natural" patients. While all nurses have the skills, not all have the right personality or easygoing nature. Unmedicated labors require a nurse to have a certain level of flexibility, competency, confidence, and patience.

Rumor has it that nurses prefer patients with epidurals because they're supposedly easier to take care of. That's not exactly true. Getting patients ready for and through the epidural process is a lot of work. Once they're comfortable, they don't always need as much interpersonal, one-to-one physical care and personal support during active labor, usually because they're relaxed and sleeping. They require a ton of monitoring, charting, and attention to detail, however, and when it's pushing time our physical workload with an epiduralized patient ramps way up. That's when we have to lift legs, turn patients, and do a lot of physical labor. Working with a well-prepared, unmedicated patient reduces our workload of monitoring and charting and, often, reduces pushing time. But unmedicated patients generally increase our workload in terms of interpersonal support, massages, and so on. So, natural versus epidural—it all balances out as far as our workload goes. Bottom line: We like natural patients. We really do.

Here's what we (hospital staff) ask of you: Come prepared to work with the hospital system (electronic fetal monitoring, frequent vital

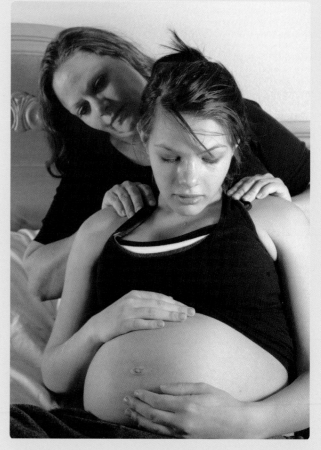

Hiring a doula can be one of the best investments you make toward having a natural birth. She is not intended to take over your partner's role, but instead to support both of you.

Many doctors, nurses, and hospital staff members actually like natural births. They're invigorating and renew our faith in a woman's ability to work with her own body.

signs, safety protocols, etc.) and bring a supply of well-established coping skills (like Lamaze, Hypno-Birthing, and someone who knows how to give a good massage). If your husband or partner, sister, mom, or friend is ready, willing, and able to provide excellent labor support—that's great. If not (and not every dad/partner is up to it), that's what your labor nurse is there for, but you might consider using a doula, too.

Hiring a doula can be one of the best investments you make in your birth experience. She's been there, knows the system, has excellent techniques, and symbolizes to the medical community that you're serious about having an unmedicated birth. Once in a while, however, an individual doula comes with a strong personal agenda and less real-world experience than she needs. Some have an idealized birth in mind that may not gel with your vision, anatomy, baby, or birth location. She may preach one style of labor preparation and look down on other techniques. Beware the doula (or friend or family member) who steps in front of your husband or partner and tries to take that person's rightful place. Most fathers want to be mom's right-hand man. A skilled doula (or labor support person) knows how to help dad be the best birthing partner he can be.

How do you find a good one? Ask around among your friends and family who've used ones they like. Contact DONA International for names of trained doulas in your area. Ask for references and make those calls. Think twice about using a doula in training or someone who wants to be a doula someday. You need one who's worked with a variety of women and had a range of birth experiences, not one who's seen a birth or two.

Make sure your doula is a good match for your partner, who has an important role in your labor process and needs to be supported during labor, too. Your doula is not meant to be a substitute for your partner. Make sure your roles are spelled out in advance. For example, maybe your doula provides medical and physical support and your partner provides emotional support. The goal is for the whole family to feel like they're enabled to experience the best birth possible.

CHOOSING AN UNMEDICATED, VAGINAL BIRTH IN A HOSPITAL

Plenty of women give birth naturally—that is, vaginally, without pain medication—in a hospital. As we noted above, though, in a hospital, "natural birth" is not necessarily the norm. Right up front, you should understand that choosing to have your birth in a hospital lowers the chances that you'll have an unmedicated, vaginal delivery. About 33 percent of all births in the United States in 2010 were Cesarean deliveries—that means that you have a one-in-three chance of ending up with a Cesarean delivery in a U.S. hospital. There are some cultural and institutional hurdles you'll face when delivering naturally in a hospital. The other challenge you might face is in your own ability to resist the urge to ask for pain medication when you're in the throes of labor. Let's face it: When you're in pain, and pain relief is within easy reach, you may be tempted to ask—or even beg!—for it.

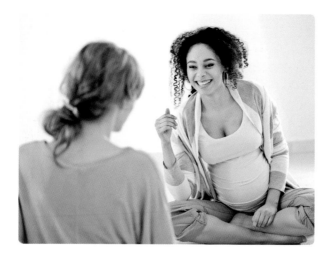

Make sure your labor support person is 100 percent on board with your natural birth plans and that she prepares for that goal during your pregnancy.

But that's not to say that it's not entirely possible to have an unmedicated, vaginal birth in a hospital. With the right plans in place, this can be a choice option for many women who want a natural childbirth experience with the peace of mind that comes from knowing that there's a safety net in the form of high-tech medical help should complications arise.

To prepare for natural childbirth in a hospital setting, you'll want to set some guidelines with yourself, your labor support team, and your health care provider about how you feel about having an unmedicated birth and what might happen if you change your mind once you're experiencing labor. Some women tell their support team up front: "Don't even mention the word 'epidural' to me!" Others give their labor partners these instructions: "Even if I beg for medication, don't give it to me!" We don't recommend the latter, because you really don't know how you and your body are going to respond to the pain of labor. And it's not fair to put your labor partners in the position of denying you relief if you're begging for their help. But we do advocate for the former—make your wishes clear up front. Set the scene that will give you the optimal chance of having the unmedicated birth that you want—whether that means asking people not to offer or suggest pain-relief medication or giving them some very specific guidelines for how you'd like them to help support you. There's a lot you can do as part of your birth plan to set the scene that will give you the optimal conditions for an unmedicated, vaginal delivery. Here are a few tips:

- Choose a health care practitioner who's supportive of natural birth.

- Ask the hospital for statistics on the percentage of births that are unmedicated, vaginal births. (If the statistics don't seem to support unmedicated, vaginal birth, find another hospital.)

- Consider working with a midwife or a doula who specializes in unmedicated, vaginal births. Studies have shown that this will increase your odds of having a drug-free, vaginal birth.

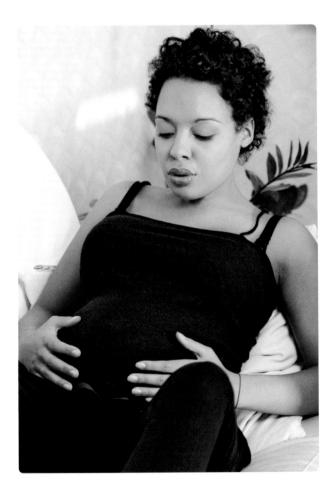

Practice natural pain-relief techniques such as breathing, meditation, and self-hypnosis during pregnancy so you'll be prepared to handle whatever labor presents to you.

- Make sure that your labor support team is 100 percent on board with your natural childbirth plan and that your support person prepares for natural childbirth with you by attending classes, reading books, and practicing natural childbirth techniques.

- Take a childbirth preparation class—such as HypnoBirthing, the Bradley Method, Lamaze, or Birthing From Within—that focuses on natural childbirth.

- Read as many books on natural childbirth as you can.

- Get online and read the birth stories of women who've successfully had an unmedicated, vaginal delivery in a hospital. Hearing firsthand accounts of women who've delivered this way will help you envision and prepare for this type of birth yourself.

- Practice natural pain-relief techniques, such as breathing, meditation, visualization, self-hypnosis, positive affirmations, massage, movement, and various labor positions (such as squats, lunges, sitting on a birthing ball, and more — see chapter 10 for a more comprehensive list).

- Find out whether you'll have access to a tub (or shower) in your labor room—many women find warm water to be one of the most soothing natural pain-management techniques.

- Find out whether your hospital routinely provides tools such as a birthing balls and "squat bars," which have been shown to help women relax their hips and work with gravity to ease the baby down the birth canal.

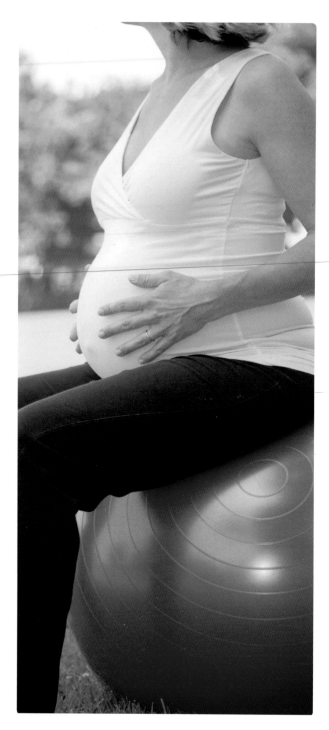

Birthing balls, like exercise balls, can help women relax their hips and work with gravity during labor. With proper instruction and supervision, they are an excellent way to prepare for your birth experience.

- Find out whether you would be required to lie on your back or stay in bed during your labor. You'll be less likely to require pain medication or labor interventions if you're free to move around and work with gravity.

- Come to the hospital equipped with the right tools to get through your labor and delivery drug free—for instance, a warm or cold compress; an iPod loaded with meditation music; massage oils; or massage tools—see chapter 10 for more ideas.

- Write out a birth plan that clearly lays out your wishes for an unmedicated, vaginal birth in a hospital—and how you plan to get there.

- Share your birth plan with your health care provider to make sure that you're all on the same page with the type of delivery you'd like to have. And then talk through the scenarios in which your health care practitioner would have to deviate from the plan for your and your baby's safety .

The Ins and Outs of Delivering in a Hospital

If you're planning to deliver in a hospital, there are a few logistical considerations to have in mind, including preadmission policies, visitor policies, check-out policies, neonatal intensive care unit (NICU) and nursery care availability, hospital-specific policies and procedures, and more.

Preadmission: Most hospitals will want you to fill out preadmission paperwork well before you go into labor. That way, when you arrive at the hospital in labor, you can focus on getting through contractions rather than on getting through paperwork. Your health care provider should be able to provide you with forms. Or ask for the appropriate forms when you take your hospital tour.

Miscellaneous hospital policies: Many hospitals have their own policies when it comes to routine procedures: what you can eat or drink during labor, who can be in the delivery room, when visitors are allowed, and more. Check with your hospital about its policies and procedures and discuss any issues with your health care provider.

NICU and nursery care: One reason why many women choose a hospital birth is that it offers access to a NICU in case of emergency, as well as around-the-clock nursery staff to help care for your newborn baby. (Not all hospitals have a NICU or twenty-four-hour nursery care, so be sure to research the services that your hospital provides.)

THE REAL DEAL: *Relax!*

Once labor begins, try to stay home as long as possible and relax if you can. Take a nap. Take a walk. Listen to music. Take a shower. If this is your first baby, you can expect to be in labor for an average of twelve hours. The more time that you can comfortably and

safely spend at home, the more likely you'll be to have a drug-free, vaginal birth. Your labor will no doubt progress more rapidly if you're feeling relaxed, in a comfortable environment. And you won't be tempted to get that epidural if it's not within easy reach! For a healthy, low-risk pregnancy, most health care providers recommend that it's time to come to the hospital when your contractions are four to five minutes apart, lasting a minute or more, for at least an hour.

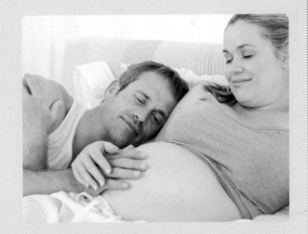

If possible, stay at home during your early labor. Pace yourself. Taking a nap, a walk, a bath, or shower will help you to relax. You'll be more comfortable and increase your chances for a natural birth if you don't come to the hospital too early.

THE REAL DEAL: *Rest!*

Many moms and dads opt to room in with their babies. This helps them bond with baby and promotes early breastfeeding, as mom can respond to baby immediately. But don't underestimate how tired you'll be from the labor and delivery. Don't be afraid to send baby to the nursery for a few hours—she'll be in good hands with the nursery staff, and you'll get to rest. If you're planning to breastfeed, be sure that the nursery staff will bring baby back to you at the first sign that she's hungry (and that they won't give baby a pacifier or formula against your wishes). Though every new mom wants to have her baby nearby, second- and third-time moms will tell you that you should accept the help and rest while you can—you won't have a nursery staff on hand at home and your body needs to rest and recuperate for the marathon of sleepless nights ahead.

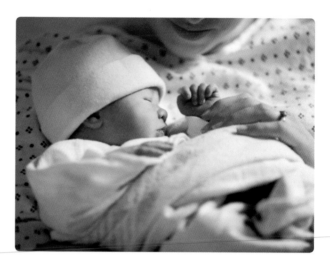

Rooming in with your baby helps parents bond, promotes breastfeeding, and helps parents learn how to care for their baby right from the start. If you're exhausted, however, don't be afraid to let baby stay in the nursery while you rest.

Labor and delivery rooms: Many hospitals now offer more comfortable, homelike settings in their labor and delivery units. Yours might offer rocking chairs, comfortable seating (and pull-out beds or cots) for labor coaches, tubs and showers, homey décor, and so on. Hospitals vary widely in terms of whether you'll stay in one room for your entire hospital stay or whether you'll be transferred to different rooms (or even different floors) for your labor, delivery, and recovery. Most hospitals offer private or semiprivate rooms, but you should ask in advance what you can expect from your own hospital. Be sure to take a tour of the facilities well in advance of your due date.

Visitor policies: Some hospitals have strict policies on visiting hours, allowing children to visit, and the number of visitors you can have. Check with your hospital to see whether it has any restrictions or requirements. And keep in mind that if your visitors are limited in number, it's usually for safety reasons, i.e., so the hospital can monitor who comes in and out of the ward, which is especially important for keeping newborn babies safe.

Check-out policies: If you've had an unmedicated, vaginal delivery, you can expect to stay at the hospital for forty-eight hours after the delivery. (And if all is well, you often have the option of leaving earlier if you choose.) Be aware that you'll have some discharge paperwork to fill out before you can leave the hospital, and that you'll need to have your baby's infant car seat with you before you'll be discharged.

Care of Mom and Baby after an Unmedicated, Vaginal Birth in a Hospital

If you're having an unmedicated, vaginal birth in a hospital, you'll most likely deliver your baby with an OB/GYN or midwife "catching" the baby and a

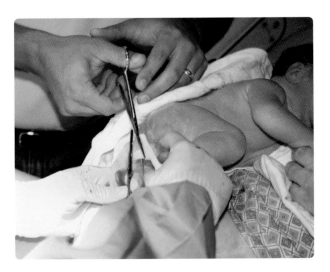

Your provider will clamp baby's umbilical cord and show your partner where to cut it if he or she should choose to take that role. Your partner might find the cord is tougher than it looks, but don't worry; you and your baby won't feel a thing!

team of nurses ready to help assess and take care of the baby in case of any complications. You can expect your health care provider to place the baby right on your chest, in your arms, immediately after the baby emerges from the birth canal. He or she may suction the baby's airways as soon as the head emerges. The baby's umbilical cord will be clamped in two places, and your partner should have the option to cut the baby's cord. A tube of blood will be collected to check the baby's blood type and for possible additional blood tests.

While the baby is lying on your chest, she'll be given an overall health assessment. An Apgar test will be done at one and five minutes after birth to assess baby's heart rate, breathing, muscle tone, reflex response, and color. As all of this is happening, your health care provider will deliver the placenta—you may hardly even notice, you'll be so busy gazing at your baby! You can usually expect baby to be weighed and measured near your bedside, and you'll be encouraged to start breastfeeding as soon as possible. Your baby will be given an ID band that matches yours and your partner's (all of the bands will be checked anytime the baby leaves the room), and your baby may be footprinted. (Tip: Bring your baby book and ask the nurse to stamp the baby book while he or she is at it!) Your baby will be wrapped in a blanket and a hat will be placed on his head to keep him warm. Within an hour after your baby's birth, he'll be given an antibiotic ointment in his eyes to prevent infection (required by law in most states), as well as an injection of vitamin K to help with blood clotting.

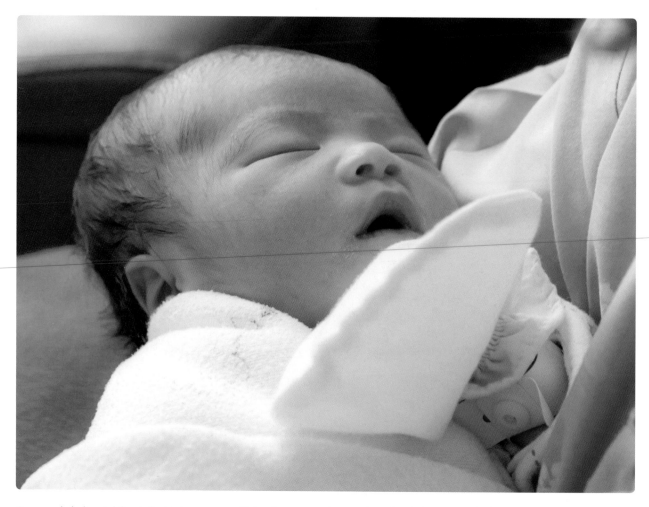

Once your baby has stabilized after birth, your nurse will clean him up, wrap him snugly, and settle him into your bed so you can rest and bond together.

If your baby needs additional care, he may be taken to an intensive care nursery. But, assuming that you and your baby are both healthy and doing well, the nurses will help you both get cleaned up and settled into bed to begin resting and bonding together. Within the first twenty-four hours of your hospital stay, your baby will have his first pediatric exam. Within forty-eight hours, your baby will have a "heel prick" test, where blood is drawn to test for certain metabolic and genetic disorders, such as phenylketonuria (PKU) and hypothyroidism (the combination of tests differs by state; the hospital staff will give you info on each test that is required and may offer other tests that are optional). You can also expect your baby to have a newborn hearing test and a hepatitis B vaccination before you leave the hospital. If you have a boy and if you choose to have him circumcised, it can be done before you leave the hospital or at your first pediatrician's visit.

THE REAL DEAL: *Knowing the Options*

About 70 percent of women get epidurals after many swore they wouldn't. That's because labor hurts more than they thought and "relief" is just one call to the anesthesiologist away. Most American women delivering in hospitals don't have many pain relief options other than natural techniques, narcotics or epidurals. Come with strategies and support for dealing with labor pain and a plan for what to do if you want to change your mind. Try something such as this nine-step approach:

1. I'll change positions or walk.

2. I'll get in the shower or tub.

3. I'll try a different breathing or relaxation technique.

4. I'll ask for massage.

5. I'll let you know if the pain is more than I can handle.

    Note: Your midwife or doctor might check your cervix and tell you you're completely dilated, and you're almost done. Or she might tell you you're 4 centimeters and have a ways to go. This information can be really valuable when planning your next steps.

6. I'll wait ten more contractions before I do anything else.

7. I'll try narcotics (if they're appropriate and safe during your stage in labor).

8. I'll start over on steps one through seven.

    Frequently all you need to get over an intense patch of labor is a plan. You might repeat steps one through seven several times and find that they're all you need. But if they're not, proceed to step nine.

9. I'll ask for an epidural and, I'll be okay with that.

    If you get an epidural, that's fine. It's a tool, just like any other labor technique, and it's there for a reason.

A Look at the Complicated Side of Childbirth

Every birth has the potential for risks and complications, and although many are screened out or diagnosed during prenatal care, some come up at the last minute. We'll cover a few common complications that arise during childbirth and how they're treated so you won't be caught by surprise.

Q. *What happens if the umbilical cord is caught around the baby's neck?*

A. While the cord being wrapped around baby's neck is often talked about like it's a huge emergency, it actually happens quite a lot, and most of the time, it's no big deal. In fact, in the majority of deliveries where the cord is around baby's neck, arm, leg, or other body part, there are no signs of it before birth and it causes no complications whatsoever.

Once baby's head has been delivered, your health care provider will slip her fingers around the neck to feel for the cord. If she feels it, she'll try to gently slip it over baby's head before she delivers the shoulders and body. If it's too tight to slip it over, she may try to let baby deliver through the loop or she'll clamp it, cut it, and unwrap it from baby's neck. Then she'll deliver the rest of baby's body, usually with no problem.

Sometimes the cord gets tugged, compressed, or pinched during labor and birth and shows up on fetal heart monitoring as the heart rate slowing down (called a deceleration). If the deceleration looks very scary, it's an indication that baby might not be getting enough circulation. In that case, if a vaginal birth isn't imminent, then a C-section might be recommended. Most of the time, these babies come out just fine and that pesky cord only adds drama to their birth story.

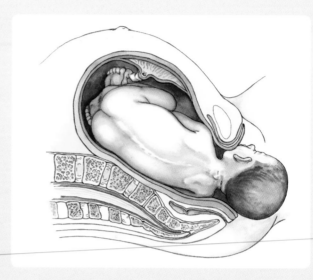

Shoulder dystocia occurs when baby's head is able to pass through the birth canal, but the shoulders get stuck because they're too big or baby is in an unnatural position.

Q. *What about shoulder dystocia?*

A. Shoulder dystocia is a term that means baby's shoulders get stuck in the birth canal after its head has been delivered. This is a very frightening situation for health care providers and mothers because when it happens, there's usually no warning. Health care providers will attempt to deliver baby as quickly as possible to avoid serious complications like fetal hypoxia (decreased oxygenation), nerve damage, broken bones (in mom and baby), maternal hemorrhage, uterine rupture, and severe perineal lacerations. In worst-case scenarios, shoulder dystocia can cause fetal death.

If your health care provider can't get baby's shoulders out by applying gentle traction, he'll call for extra help in the delivery room and do a number of maneuvers (and very quickly) to try and change baby's angle, make more space in Mom's pelvis, and hopefully, pull baby free of the birth canal.

He'll have you, your nurse, and your partner put the head of your bed down to a low position and help you pull your legs back and as wide as possible at an almost jack-knifed angle. You might need an episiotomy to make more space in your vagina, too. He'll push down hard on the area directly above your pubic bone while you push (like you did when trying to get baby's head out) with all your might. Then your provider will wedge his fingers under baby's armpit (if he can reach it) and try to maneuver baby out. You might have to roll over to an all-fours, hands and knees position.

Usually these maneuvers work, but sometimes they cause injuries (such as fracture of baby's collarbone) to mom and baby. As bad as that sounds, these kinds of minor injuries generally heal quickly and are much better than the dire consequences of being stuck. If your provider is not able to get baby out vaginally, then you'll be having an emergency C-section.

Though shoulder dystocia is among the scariest birth complications, it's also fairly uncommon. The overall incidence of shoulder dystocia occurs in 0.6 to 1.4 percent of babies between 5 pounds, 8 ounces and 8 pounds, 13 ounces (2.5 and 4 kg). If baby weighs more than that, the rate increases to between 5 and 9 percent.

Q. What happens if baby is malpositioned?

A. The term malpositioned can mean a lot of different things. It might indicate baby is breech or in a side-lying (transverse) position or that she's head down, but with her face looking up toward mom's abdomen instead of down at mom's bottom. It might also mean baby's facing the right direction, but her head is turned just a little to the side.

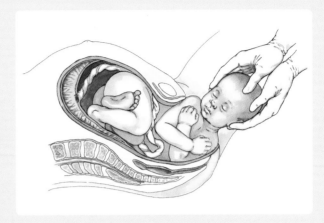

In a normal birth, shoulders slide out right after the delivery of baby's head.

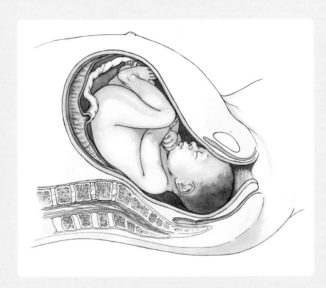

In an occiput posterior position, a baby's head is down, but he's facing mom's abdomen instead of being occiput anterior—facing mom's bottom; the most common and easiest position for a vaginal birth.

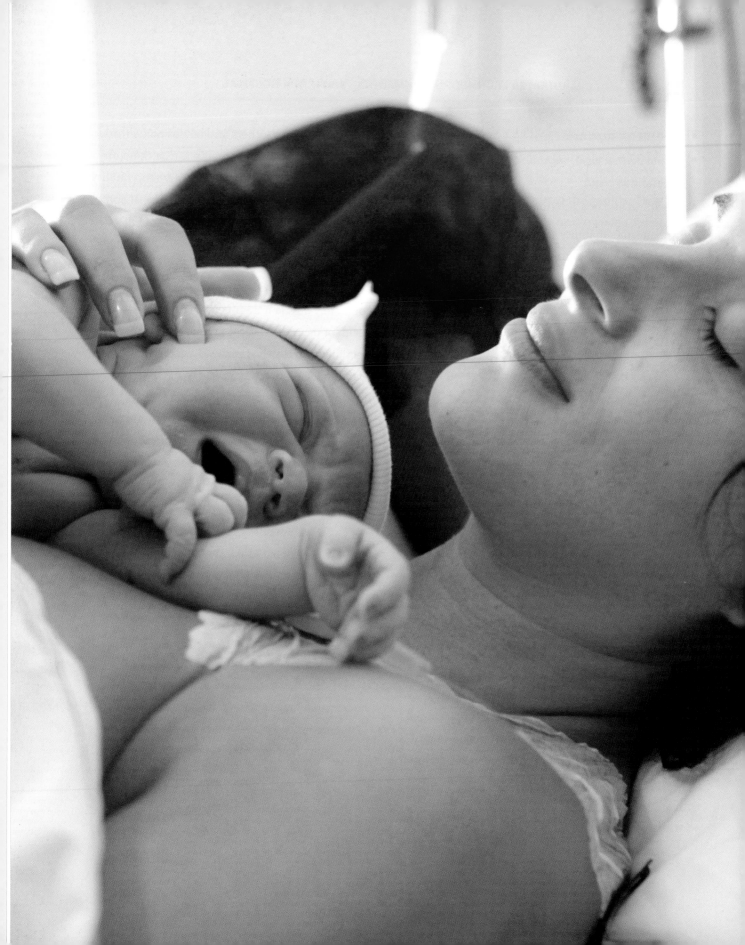

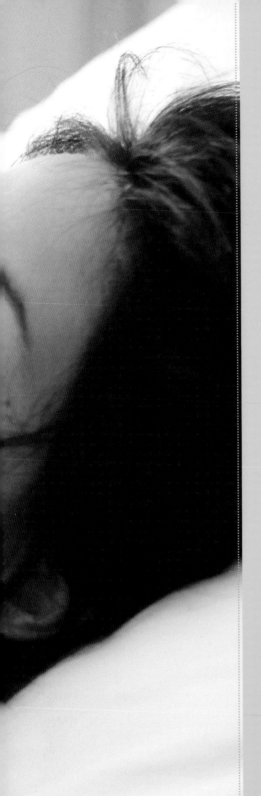

CHAPTER 5

Epidural, Vaginal Birth in a Hospital

What it is, why it may or may not be right for you, pros and cons, and how to prepare for this labor path

Almost all women deliver their babies in hospitals. About 68 percent will have vaginal deliveries, and most will have an epidural. It is so common to deliver vaginally with an epidural and so widely available and culturally accepted that many women consider it the normal way to give birth.

Getting an epidural during labor and birth is the most common pain management technique used for vaginal deliveries and C-sections. In fact, about 71 percent of American women get epidurals. In other parts of the world, epidural use varies, depending on what other pain relief options are available, cultural norms, availability of trained anesthetists/anesthesiologists, and other factors. Epidurals are considered to be safe and effective at eliminating what most women and their health care providers consider severe pain.

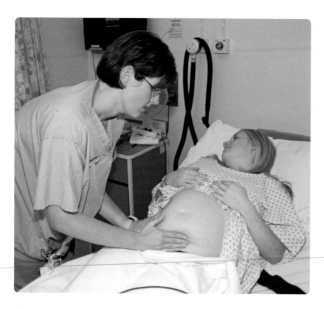

Have a wait-and-see attitude before making the choice to have an epidural. Your support team will help guide you in the right direction for your particular circumstances.

Here's what the American Congress of Obstetricians and Gynecologists and the American Society of Anesthesiologists say about pain relief in labor:

"Labor causes severe pain for many women. There is no other circumstance where it is considered acceptable for an individual to experience untreated severe pain, amenable to safe intervention, while under a physician's care. In the absence of a medical contraindication, maternal request is a sufficient medical indication for pain relief during labor. Pain management should be provided whenever medically indicated. Of the various pharmacologic methods used for pain relief during labor and delivery, neuraxial analgesia techniques (epidural, spinal, and combined spinal–epidural) are the most flexible, effective, and least depressing to the central nervous system, allowing for an alert participating woman and an alert neonate."

WHO GETS EPIDURALS?

Women who receive epidurals generally fall into one of three camps:

- Women who planned on having a natural labor but ultimately chose an epidural when labor proved more challenging than anticipated
- Women who weren't committed to any particular pain management technique during pregnancy but intended to keep their options open
- Women who knew from the start that an epidural was the only way to go as far as they were concerned

It's unclear exactly how many women who intend to have a natural birth change their mind during labor and opt for an epidural. Those of us who work with laboring women know, however, it's a very common scenario, especially for first-time mothers. That's because first labors tend to last longer than subsequent labors and many first-time mothers underestimate how challenging contractions can be. When they run out of energy or motivation to continue using natural techniques, many ask for IV pain management (a shot of narcotics). When that doesn't last long enough or work well enough, their only other option is an epidural.

Occasionally an epidural will be recommended by a midwife or doctor as a tool to help stalled labor progress, to allow a provider to manually rotate or reposition a malpositioned baby, use a vacuum extractor or forceps, or for some other medical reason, even when mom is managing contractions quite well using natural techniques.

Making the decision to switch gears from all-natural labor to an epidural is sometimes emotionally difficult. Some women feel like they've failed if they opt for an epidural, like they didn't try hard enough or weren't devoted enough to their natural techniques. Many wait so long to access pain relief that they're exhausted and emotionally distraught. Still others feel like they have to go against their partner's wishes, when that person is more invested in a natural birth than the mother herself.

The vast majority of women who choose to get an epidural are greatly relieved. Many wonder why they were so resistant to getting one in the first place. There are a few women who dislike the way their epidural makes them feel or associate their epidural with subsequent complications, leaving them unhappy they chose this option. Some women find it unsettling when they can't feel their legs. Most, however, are very happy when the epidural kicks in and the pain is over.

For women who were neither for nor against epidurals going in to labor, making the choice to get one may be less challenging. These women face labor with a wait-and-see attitude. Once they understand how labor will affect them, they may try narcotics first or may go straight for an epidural. Again, most women who choose to get an epidural are greatly relieved and happy they made this choice.

For some women, labor without an epidural is unthinkable. They approach labor much like they would a root canal, surgery, or other potentially painful experience. They know it's going to hurt and don't want anything to do with the pain. Although some opt to get their epidural before labor

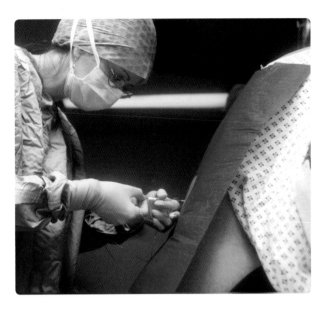

An anesthetist or anesthesiologist administers epidurals with a sterile technique to place tubing into a fluid-filled space near the spinal cord. After, she administers pain medications through that tubing, and labor pain subsides.

gets painful, the majority of women wait until their contractions are regular and their cervix is dilating before they have the epidural placed.

Many women choose to get epidurals because it's the only pain management option that takes away most or all of the pain associated with labor and birth. Other options may dial it down and make contractions tolerable, but an epidural can potentially turn the pain off. Once women understand how painful labor can be for them (it's a subjective experience and feels more or less painful to individual women), they decide to use the best pain management tool available.

Pros and Cons of a Vaginal Delivery with an Epidural

Pros

- An epidural can take away the pain of labor, helping you to relax and enjoy the experience of giving birth, while allowing you to be fully mentally alert and present for your baby's birth.

- An epidural can allow you and your partner to rest—and even sleep—through some of the long hours of labor.

- Epidurals have been widely used and generally proven safe for mom and baby.

Cons

- An epidural usually requires having a bladder catheter inserted and continuous electronic fetal monitoring, which generally necessitate confining a laboring woman to bed.

- Occasionally an epidural won't work properly to provide enough pain relief, so an epidural may need to be readjusted or replaced.

- An epidural can cause complications such as a drop in blood pressure (which is treated by changing the mother's position, administering oxygen, and giving intravenous fluid).

- An epidural can cause an abnormal heart rate in the fetus (generally related to the changes that occur in the mother). This, again, may require changing the mother's position, administering oxygen, giving intravenous fluids, trying to stop or decrease the number and intensity of contractions, or rarely, doing an emergency delivery.

- Many women feel too numb to push, which can make pushing less effective.

- Some women may experience shivering or itching with an epidural (these are normal side effects of narcotics, not specific to epidurals).

- An epidural may make you feel "numb" to—that is, detached from—the actual experience of giving birth.

- An epidural can slow down labor for some women, requiring the administration of Pitocin.

- Some women are surprised that their epidural may be turned down at the pushing stages and that they have to work to push their baby out at the end.

- Some women have difficulty walking for up to several hours after giving birth because they're still feeling the effects of their epidurals.

- Some women may experience backache or headache for several hours to days after having an epidural.

- In rare cases, an epidural can cause complications such as residual numbness, nerve injury at the needle insertion site, respiratory distress, paralysis, brain damage, or death.

- Some studies have shown that babies born to mothers who had epidurals may have some initial trouble latching on for breastfeeding and may have some short-term neurobehavioral effects, including irritability and a decreased ability to track an object visually. (This is not always true, and wanting to breastfeed is not a reason in itself to decline an epidural.)

HOW TO PREPARE FOR A VAGINAL BIRTH WITH AN EPIDURAL

If you would like to have a vaginal birth with an epidural in a hospital, you can prepare yourself ahead of time for the experience by doing the following:

- Take a childbirth education class—even if you know you want an epidural. A class will give you a general overview of what to expect during childbirth, making you a more confident, informed participant in your own birth. Ask around to find a class in your area that covers epidurals as part of the course material, so you'll know what to expect. And keep in mind that it's still a good idea to learn about natural techniques for managing pain to help get you through the early stages of labor before you get your epidural. Also, you'll be prepared in case you change your mind about getting an epidural, if your epidural doesn't work, or if you can't get epidural after all. (What if there's no anesthesiologist available? What if you get to the hospital too late? Best to be prepared.)

- Go online and read the birth stories of women who've had vaginal deliveries with epidurals in a hospital. Reading these firsthand accounts will help you envision and prepare for this type of birth yourself. You may even want to watch a few videos of an epidural being inserted, so you'll know what to expect. (Go to YouTube and search on keywords such as "epidural for childbirth.")

- Talk to your partner, labor coach, and/or labor support team about your plans for having an epidural and include it in your birth plan.

- Talk to friends who've delivered their babies with epidurals. Get their take on what the experience was like.

- Be sure to take a tour of your hospital so you can see the facilities firsthand, meet the staff, and ask any specific questions that you might have. Ask your hospital for any statistics they can provide on vaginal deliveries at the hospital in recent years. See whether it's possible to meet with and talk to the anesthesiologists who routinely perform epidurals at your hospital. If you have medical issues, your doctor or midwife might want you to formally consult with the anesthesiologist during your last trimester. That way, you can discuss your history in a calm, controlled setting, instead of when you are contracting every two minutes.

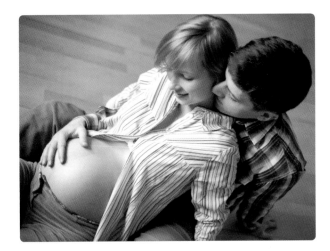

Take a childbirth education class, even if you are planning on having an epidural. You'll learn what it's like to have one, how to cope with labor beforehand, and how to prepare in case you don't get one in time.

- Talk to your health care provider about the process for getting an epidural and any concerns you might have. Share your birth plan with your health care provider to make sure you agree on the type of delivery you'd like to have. And then talk through the scenarios in which your health care practitioner would have to deviate from your plan for the safety of mom and baby.

WHAT YOU NEED TO KNOW ABOUT EPIDURALS

An epidural is a specific type of pain management system that eliminates labor and childbirth pain. The American Pregnancy Association describes it in this way:

> "Epidural anesthesia is regional anesthesia that blocks pain in a particular region of the body. The goal of an epidural is to provide analgesia, or pain relief, rather than complete anesthesia, which is total lack of feeling. Epidurals block the nerve impulses from the lower spinal segments, resulting in decreased sensation in the lower half of the body. Epidural medications fall into a class of drugs called local anesthetics, such as bupivacaine, chloroprocaine, or lidocaine. They are often delivered in combination with opioids or narcotics, such as fentanyl and sufentanil, to decrease the required dose of local anesthetic. This way pain relief is achieved with minimal effects. These medications may be used in combination with epinephrine, fentanyl, morphine, or clonidine to prolong the epidural's effect or stabilize the mother's blood pressure."

Epidurals last for as long as they're needed because once an epidural catheter (tube) has been inserted into your spinal cord area, it can administer a continuous dose of numbing medication for an indefinite period of time. It can also be used to provide pain management for surgery in case the patient needs a C-section. Once it's no longer needed, the tube is removed and the medication gradually wears off over the course of a couple of hours.

Preparing for an Epidural

Epidurals are administered by registered nurses or doctors with advanced training in anesthesia. Many hospitals employ certified registered nurse anesthetists (CRNAs) to administer epidurals and provide anesthesia for C-sections and other surgical procedures. Some hospitals use anesthesiologists (medical doctors), and still others have a combination of the two.

Once a patient decides she wants an epidural, a few things must happen before she can get one. She has to be formally admitted to the hospital (which usually takes a couple of phone calls and some paperwork). Her doctor has to order the procedure, and consent forms have to be signed. An IV must be started and lab work drawn. The patient has to receive at least one-half to one full liter of IV fluid (usually a solution called Lactated Ringer's) before she receives an epidural. Epidural medication causes blood vessel dilation, which can dramatically lower mom's blood pressure. That

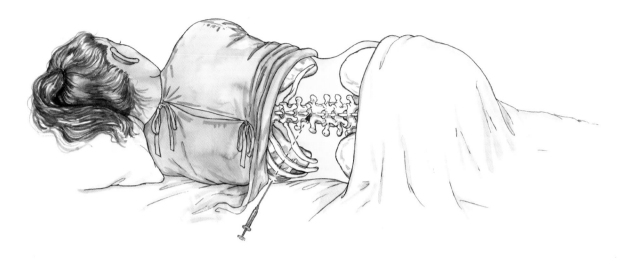

Patient in a side-lying position with an exposed area indicating where on the spine an epidural would be placed.

can cause baby's heart rate to drop as well as cause mom to experience dizziness, nausea, and vomiting. To prevent that from happening, IV fluids are always administered prior to epidural administration. When there is extra fluid circulation in the blood vessels, blood pressure usually stays within the normal range.

Once these preparations are under way, the nurse will call the anesthetist. In many big hospitals, the anesthetist is already on duty and in the labor and delivery department and usually available within a very short period of time. In some smaller hospitals, he or she has to be called in from somewhere outside the hospital (though the location shouldn't be more than twenty minutes away), and the patient has to wait for an anesthitist to arrive.

After the anesthetist arrives in the patient's room, she'll consult with the patient about her health history and educate the patient about the pros and cons and potential risks, benefits, and complications associated with epidurals. One way to make the pre-epidural consultation move more quickly and smoothly (especially if you have a complicated history or specific concerns) is to schedule a consultation before you go into labor. The anesthetist can take your medical history, talk about pros and cons, and then when you come into the hospital in labor, they already know you.

Once all these preprocedure preparations are made, the nurse will help her patient get in the right position to receive her epidural. Some anesthetists want their patient to sit on the side of the bed, and others want her to lie on her side. This is entirely up to the anesthetist and is based on how she was trained, the patient's size and anatomy, and the situation. The patient will pull her knees up (if she's on her side), curl up around her belly, and push her back out. Some anesthetists describe the position as like "a shrimp on a cocktail glass" or like "an angry cat." The idea is to expose the back and create space between spinal discs.

The anesthetist will open his supplies and equipment, being careful to keep everything sterile. The nurse will place a blood pressure cuff and a pulse oximeter (like a curved barrette that gently clamps onto a patient's finger or toe to measure her heart rate and oxygen saturation) on her patient and make sure the IV is still running smoothly.

Then the anesthetist will scrub an area about waist height on the patient's back, using a special cleaning solution. He'll tape a sterile paper and plastic shield around his "work area" and prepare to administer a numbing shot to the patient's skin. This local anesthetic is usually the only part of getting an epidural that hurts. It's very similar to getting novocaine at the dentist, and it will sting and burn for about ten seconds. Once that injection takes effect, he'll administer a second, deeper shot to numb the area further. That second shot doesn't normally hurt as much as the first one did. The rest of the procedure is usually described as feeling uncomfortable or weird but not painful. If it hurts, speak up and your anesthetist will give you more numbing medication or try a different technique or location.

Receiving an Epidural

Once your skin is numb, the anesthetist is ready to put in the epidural tube. The patient will be encouraged to curl up as best as she can and hold still. Many patients are worried they won't be able to do this, but virtually all of them do. They're motivated to get out of pain and cautious about making any

sudden moves that might injure their spine. Surprisingly few women move so much that the anesthetist can't do his job. When that does happen, some women receive a narcotic pain shot (like fentanyl) in their IV to relax them. If that's not enough or a woman can't get herself under control (this happens rarely), the anesthetist will decline to do the procedure. As mentioned, most women show a lot more control than they ever thought they could, and most anesthetists are very adept at hitting a moving target (e.g., a laboring woman in pain).

The needle used to put in the epidural is relatively long. We don't usually recommend that husbands/partners watch this part of the procedure because some are disturbed at the size of the needle. Some anesthetists refuse to administer epidurals if there are any visitors in the room because their reactions are distracting and might interfere with his ability to do a good job. It's important that the anesthetist maintain sterile technique while putting in an epidural. That can be more difficult when there are many people in the room. Once in a while patients are upset when their visitors are sent from the room, but most understand that their nurse will be there to support them and their anesthetist needs total concentration. If it means they'll be out of pain faster, most are fine with that.

The anesthetist will push the needle (which encases a tiny catheter) between two spinal discs. He'll advance it slowly until he feels a loss of resistance. It's a blind procedure (you can't see where the needle goes once it's past the skin) that's done by touch. The anesthetist gets a feeling for when he's in the right spot, then tests it by injecting a small amount of air through a syringe. His needle does not pierce the spinal cord but instead goes to a fluid-filled area outside the spinal cord. Once he knows he's in the right spot, he'll pull back on the syringe to check for blood or spinal fluid. If there isn't any of either, then he'll give a test dose of medication. The nurse will then start watching the patient's pulse rate carefully. If it speeds up, it indicates the needle is in a blood vessel and has to be pulled back. If the pulse remains steady, that means it's safe to remove the needle, leave the catheter in place, and inject the medication that will make the patient numb.

The nurse will take frequent blood pressures (every few minutes for a while, followed by every fifteen minutes), and the anesthetist will tape the catheter securely. Many patients worry the catheter will come out when they lie on it or squirm in bed. This rarely happens, because the anesthetist uses a lot of tape to hold it in place. Plus, very few patients do much rolling or squirming once their pain is gone and their legs are numb.

It might take up to twenty minutes—though it's usually a lot less—for the pain to go away. You might feel like each contraction is a little shorter and less intense than the one before. Soon your nurse might ask, "How did that contraction feel?" and your answer will be "What contraction?" For the majority of patients, the pain will be almost entirely eliminated.

The catheter will be hooked up to an IV pump and a bag of solution that will administer a continuous dose of numbing medicine. If the patient begins to feel pain and she's not ready to deliver, the anesthetist (and sometimes the patient herself,

depending on how the epidural is set up) can administer an extra dose (called a bolus) into the catheter. The catheter stays in place until the patient and her health care providers decide she no longer needs it.

The needle used to put in the epidural is relatively long. We don't usually recommend that husbands/partners watch this part of the procedure because some are disturbed at the size of the needle.

Start to finish, getting an epidural might take up to an hour or longer. If the pain is severe, your nurse might recommend IV medication to make the wait and the procedure more tolerable, but patients should come into labor with the understanding that epidurals aren't instant. They can't be rushed. No one can take shortcuts. Every part of the procedure is essential to make your epidural safe and effective. That's one of the reasons why all labor patients should take prenatal education classes and study a few natural pain management techniques.

When an Epidural Doesn't Work the First Time

Occasionally epidurals don't work as intended. If the catheter runs along only one side of the nerves that supply the uterus and legs, mom might get one-sided pain relief or have a "window" of pain. When that happens, the anesthetist can sometimes pull back on the catheter (just a tiny bit). If that doesn't work, the epidural will have to be removed and re-placed. The procedure has to go through the same steps every time, but since you already have your IV and your skin might already be numb, the procedure might go more smoothly the second time. Typically, the second epidural works well with no further complications.

What if your anesthetist can't get the epidural in right? If she's having a tough time, it might not be because she's inex-perienced or unskilled, but because you have a challenging back or aren't in an ideal position. Give her the benefit of the doubt and let her try twice. If you need a third attempt, you're entirely justified in asking for another anesthetist. What if there isn't another anesthetist? Then you have to choose just how much you want an epidural.

The Types of Epidurals

There are a few varieties of epidurals, but they all work roughly the same. Here's a rundown of some commonly used epidural terms:

Standard epidural, a.k.a. regional epidural. After the epidural catheter is in place, a combination of medications (narcotics such as fentanyl and anes-thetics) is administered through a pump or repeated injections. The abdomen, back, pelvis, vagina, legs, and feet might all feel numb. The heavy, "dead-leg" feeling below the thighs might last for only the first hour. The pain caused by contractions and the baby pushing through the birth canal, however, should be reduced to almost none. Anesthetists say that the goal of an epidural isn't to take the pain completely away (though most patients disagree with that), but to make it tolerable. They say that if it reduces pain to a 2 or 3 on a scale of 1 to 10, then it's doing a good job. Most patients, however, say their pain level after getting an epidural is 0 or 1.

A combined spinal-epidural (CSE) is the same as above, but an initial, fast-acting dose of pain-relieving medication is injected into the intrathe-cal space (the outermost membrane covering the spinal cord) and the epidural space. Then the needle is pulled back and the catheter is advanced into the epidural space. Sometimes this initial dose of medication lasts long enough that further medication doesn't need to be infused through the catheter. It works quickly, but without the "dead leg" feeling associated with a standard epidural. If more medication is needed later, it can be infused through the epidural catheter. The benefit is its fast pain-relieving action that leaves patients more able to move their legs and change positions. It's not as appropriate, however, when labor is expected to last a long time because the anesthetist cannot "test" the epidural catheter to make sure it's working.

Other terms:

- **Light epidural:** This means that the epidural takes the edge off the pain but leaves the patient able to feel pressure and move her legs. She might also feel some of the pain of contractions.

THE REAL DEAL: *Get in Line!*

Epidurals are given on a first-come, first-served basis, but emergencies always get to cut in line. If you're in labor at the same time as many other women and there aren't enough anesthetists to go around, you might have to wait a while before it's your turn. It's not like taking a number at the deli, though. There are many factors to consider when scheduling which patient will get her epidural before others. For example, a woman who is speeding through labor might need to get hers before a patient in early labor. A patient who needs an emergency C-section goes straight to the front of the line. A patient who is in desperate pain might get hers before a patient who is managing better. Most patients don't have to wait very long, and staff members aren't trying to play favorites or make you suffer. They're just taking care of more than one mother at a time.

What can you do if you're in pain and have to wait? Try changing positions, getting in a tub, asking for a massage, or for IV pain medication. Take a peek at chapter 4 for other tips on how to have a hospital birth without an epidural.

What if there's no time to get an epidural? It sometimes happens that babies are born before a patient can get her epidural. Don't ask hospital staff to take shortcuts, because administering a safe epidural is a very precise process. Plus, you can count your blessings that your labor was quick!

- **Heavy epidural:** This means the patient doesn't feel anything below the waist. She can't move her legs, change positions, or feel any sensations in her uterus or vagina.
- **Bolus:** This is an extra dose of numbing medication given through the epidural catheter if her initial or continuous dose isn't providing enough relief.

You can ask for a specific type of epidural, but your anesthetist is going to do the procedure her own way in the manner she thinks will provide the best, most appropriate pain relief. Some of the effects of epidural medication are unpredictable. The same dose given to one patient may deliver a "heavy" effect, while on another, it's "light." One patient might be speeding through labor, while another is plodding along and needs an epidural for many hours. Try not to have too many demands or expectations about your epidural. This is a job best left to the anesthetist.

HOW AN EPIDURAL AFFECTS YOUR LABOR

Following an epidural, your labor will be a whole lot less painful. You probably won't feel your contractions, or if you do, they won't feel like pain. Some women say they feel pressure or movement, but not pain. You may or may not be able to move your legs. You'll almost certainly not be able to walk or get out of bed. Your nurse and labor support people will help you turn from side to side occasionally and help you change positions. If you've been in labor for a while or were in a lot of pain before getting an epidural, you might feel very tired and sleepy once the pain is gone. You should be able to sleep (although the epidural medication won't cause you to become sleepy).

What about going to the bathroom? You'll get up to the bathroom and empty your bladder right before your epidural is administered. After that, you won't be able to get up to urinate. If you feel the need (and most women don't) to urinate or feel pain in your bladder area, tell your nurse. She might recommend that you try to use a bedpan. Depending on how dense your epidural is (how numb you are), you might not be able to go and you might not feel like you need to. That's why every few hours (more or less), your nurse will drain your bladder with a catheter. Many women hate the idea of having a catheter because they think it will hurt. Don't worry. You're numb down there and won't feel it.

Your nurse doesn't want to insert a catheter more than two or three times during labor, because every time she puts one through the urethra it increases risks of introducing bacteria and causing infection. If your bladder needs to be drained too many times, she might put in a Foley catheter that stays in the bladder until you have the baby. Different hospitals have different catheter guidelines, and some might put in a Foley catheter right away. Others won't. Just go with your health care provider's recommendations. The catheter will be taken out before the baby is born, and you'll be able to go to the bathroom once your epidural wears off.

What about pushing? Some women feel increased pain when they're fully dilated and as the baby is pushing through the birth canal. Many women, however, can't feel a thing. Your nurse will monitor your contractions and your baby's heart rate, watching for certain patterns that indicate you're progressing toward second stage labor. She'll also check your cervix occasionally to monitor dilation. When you're completely dilated (10 cm), she'll assess your ability to push and how low in the birth canal your baby has descended. She'll help you get into a good pushing position (which depends on how well you can move), help you pull your legs back (or show your family how to support them), and teach you an effective pushing technique. If you can't feel when to push, she'll tell you when you're contracting and coach you through the pushing process, step-by-step.

Once in a while, a patient is just too numb to push effectively. When that happens, sometimes the best thing to do is to allow the baby and uterus to do most of the work. This process is sometimes called "laboring down." Once the baby moves as low as she can go in the birth canal without mom's help, then the patient will start actively pushing the baby out. Sometimes the epidural has to be allowed to wear off enough that the patient can feel when to push, control her own movements, and be actively involved in the pushing process.

Potential Side Effects and Complications from an Epidural

- Nausea—about 20 to 30 percent of women who receive epidurals are affected.

- Itching—about 30 to 50 percent of women may experience itching.

- Fever—can affect about 20 percent of women. Often the physician cannot determine whether the fever is from the epidural or an infection in the amniotic fluid and therefore has to assume that there may be an infection in the amniotic fluid, which necessitates treating the woman with antibiotics.

- Hypotension—a drop in maternal blood pressure that could affect the baby; this occurs more with higher doses of medication. With proper treatment, this should not harm the mother or the baby.

- Severe headache—can be caused by a leakage of spinal fluid, usually affecting less than 1 percent of women, but can last for several days and is also treatable.

- Other potential but rare side effects include the following: Infection, bleeding, nerve damage, shivering, ringing of the ears, backache, soreness where the needle is inserted, or difficulty urinating (this can also be a side effect of just having a baby). Some women may have difficulty walking for a few hours after birth, as the lower half of their body may still feel numb. Seizures and even death may occur if pain medication is accidentally injected directly into the bloodstream.

EPIDURAL FAQS

Q. *Will an epidural harm my baby?*

A. Any pain relief medication you take will cross the placenta and reach the baby. Though this is a topic of continued study, most research has shown that the baby absorbs only a small amount of the medicine, which has not been known to cause any harm. Epidurals are widely regarded as safe for both mom and baby. Of course, as with any medical procedure, complications can occur. And some studies suggest that babies may have trouble latching on after delivery, which can lead to breastfeeding difficulties. Other studies suggest that the baby may experience respiratory depression, fetal malpositioning, and nonreassuring changes in the fetal heart rate, which may increase the need for forceps, vacuum, Cesarean deliveries, and episiotomies.

Q. *How soon can I get an epidural?*

A. The American Congress of Obstetricians and Gynecologists states that the indication for epidural is pain, so you can technically get an epidural as soon as you and your health care provider think you're ready for one. Some hospitals encourage women to wait until they're at least 4 centimeters dilated because they want to be sure that you're in true labor and that labor won't be stalled by giving an epidural too early. (If this happens, you may be given the medicine Pitocin to help speed up labor.) But it really depends on the situation. The main thing is that the laboring woman is in pain, she is requesting an epidural, and she and her health care provider are committed to delivery.

Q. *I'm terrified of needles. Is getting an epidural going to hurt?*

A. We're not going to lie. Getting an epidural can feel pretty uncomfortable. But trust us, it's nothing compared to the pain you may be feeling from contractions—and you'll feel relief within minutes. You may find that you're so grateful for the pain relief that an epidural brings that you'll be offering to name the baby after your anesthesiologist! In short, most women would agree that the procedure involved in getting an epidural hurts far less than the contractions themselves.

Q. *If I have an epidural, am I more likely to end up with a C-section?*

A. Studies show that epidurals actually do not increase the C-section rate. They do, however, seem to increase the rate of operative vaginal birth, where a vacuum or forceps might be used to help extract the baby.

Q. *Can I take a wait-and-see approach before deciding on whether to get an epidural?*

A. Of course. Nobody knows what her labor is going to be like until she is actually experiencing it. It's good to keep an open mind. Just be aware that at some point, your health care provider may say that it's too late to get an epidural, as you'll be pushing very soon, and it would be too difficult to place an epidural at that point. Also, the pain medication may not even have time to take effect before your baby is out! Typically it's too late to get an epidural when you are (roughly) less than one hour away from birth. Usually that's when you are fully dilated (10 cm), though it can be sooner than that if your labor is moving very quickly. In general, the ideal time to get an epidural is between 4 and 8 centimeters. That way, you can be relatively sure that you are in active labor, but you also aren't ready to start pushing soon. That being said, there are many situations in which epidurals are given on either side of that range. Sometimes women are fully dilated (10 centimeters) and get epidurals. Nothing is absolute—everyone's labor is a little different.

Q. *What if I don't get to the hospital in time to get an epidural?*
A. It happens, and it's okay. Labor nurses, midwives, and doctors all deliver babies in circumstances with and without pain medication. They will help you and talk you through it. Generally this only happens when you are so close to delivery that the time it takes to push out the baby is shorter than the time it takes to get an epidural and have it give you pain relief. Otherwise what would happen is that you would arrive at the hospital, push your baby out, and then have the option for some pain medication postpartum. The good news is that if you don't get an epidural, you'll most likely be able to get right up after birth, and even have a shower if you'd like.

Most women would agree that the procedure involved in getting an epidural hurts far less than the contractions themselves.

Inside Information

Some patients come into labor with a list of specific requests. "I'll have a light epidural. I don't want to feel any pain, but make sure I can still move my legs." Getting an epidural is significantly more difficult than making a latte. You can't really order off the menu. The type of epidural you receive depends on many factors: what stage of labor you're in, your anesthetist's training and technique, your anatomy and response to medications, how long you might need your epidural, whether you might need to have a C-section, and even how busy things are on the labor unit. Once you've made the choice to have an epidural, talk to the anesthetist about it and then go with his or her best recommendations. Once you've read the description in this chapter about how epidurals are inserted, you'll understand a little better why they're not custom-ordered, but they're not one-size-fits-all, either.

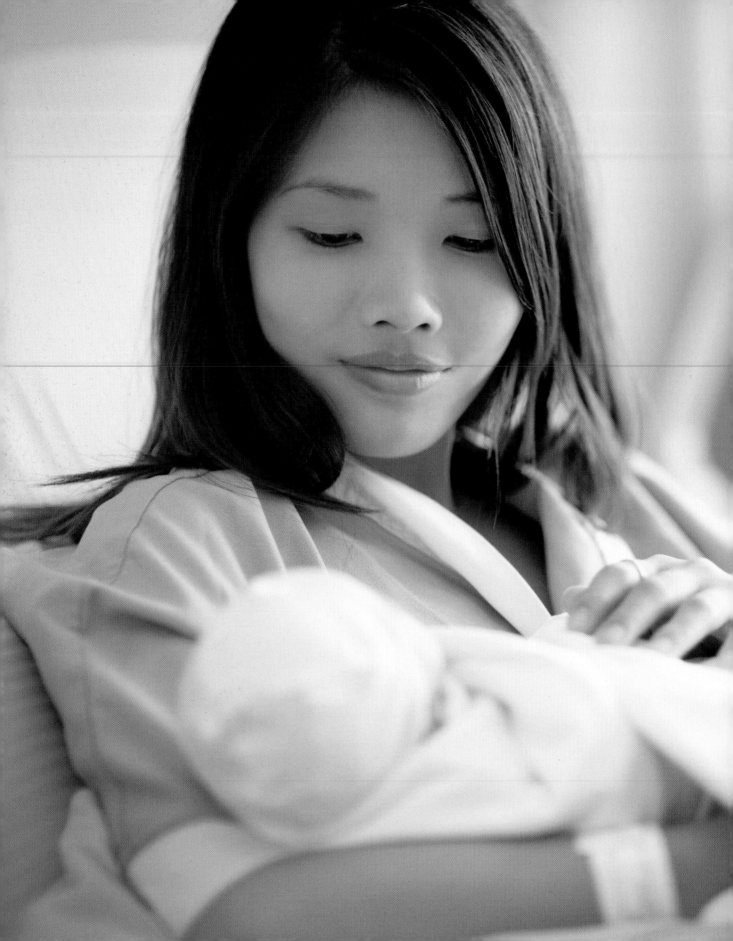

CHAPTER 6

Induction of Labor in a Hospital

What it is, why it may or may not be right for you, pros and cons, and how to prepare for this labor path

If you're nearing the end of your pregnancy and you develop a complication, such as high blood pressure or severe gestational diabetes, your health care provider may decide that it would be safer to deliver your baby than to wait for labor to kick in on its own. In such instances, your health care provider may recommend an induction—a way to naturally or artificially stimulate labor. (We'll talk more about the range of ways that labor might be induced later in this chapter.) Induction can be an important, lifesaving tool if a situation arises where your baby might have a greater chance of thriving outside, rather than inside, the womb.

Induction also happens for nonmedical reasons. We'll talk more about medical versus nonmedical ("elective") reasons for induction in this chapter.

In recent years, the practice of induction has come under a great deal of scrutiny—especially for inductions performed before 39 weeks—as more inductions were being routinely performed for nonmedical reasons and as more studies have shown that having labor induced increases the odds that you'll need further medical interventions or a C-section. One such study, published in the July 2010 issue of the journal *Obstetrics & Gynecology*, showed that among women giving birth for the first time, those who had their labor induced were two to three times more likely to have a C-section than those who went into labor naturally.

All deliveries, whether induced or not, have some inherent risks, and it's important for you and your health care provider to weigh the risks and benefits of your own unique situation when determining whether to induce labor.

MEDICAL REASONS FOR INDUCTION

There are many reasons why your health care provider might recommend an induction, including some of the following:

- You've gone two weeks beyond your due date and your health care provider has determined that it would put the baby at risk to wait longer (because your placenta may start to deteriorate or because the baby is getting so large that delivery might become more difficult). Some health care providers will want to induce if you've reached 42 weeks, while others will want to induce closer to 41 weeks if the cervix is more open and ripe, as some data has shown that inducing closer to 41 weeks can decrease the risk of late fetal demise.

- Your baby is not growing properly, and your health care provider has determined that it would be safer to deliver the baby than to take a wait-and-see approach.

- You're having complications toward the end of your pregnancy and your health care provider thinks that it would be safest to deliver the baby right away. These complications include, but are not limited to:

  - Hypertension (high blood pressure), diabetes, or other chronic medical conditions that might be putting you or your baby at risk

  - Lower-than-normal levels of amniotic fluid (*oligohydramnios*)

  - Your placenta is beginning to deteriorate, potentially depriving your baby of nutrients and oxygen.

  - Your water has broken, but your labor isn't progressing. (Most health care providers will want to induce labor six to twenty-four hours after your water has broken, depending on the situation; some birth centers will wait up to forty-eight hours, but the patients are strictly monitored.)

Nonmedical Reasons for Induction

There are times when an induction will be scheduled for nonmedical reasons, such as:

- Mom has a history of superfast labors or lives a long way from the hospital and wants to be sure she gets to the labor unit in time.
- Dad is being deployed and wants to be at his child's birth.
- There's no child care available for other children, unless she arranges it in advance and schedules an induction.

Though these aren't ideal reasons for mom to be induced, they do represent compelling reasons why induction might be a good idea. Discuss the risks and benefits with your provider and decide what fits with your circumstances.

Consider These Risk Factors

You're not a good candidate for induction if:

- You've had a prior C-section or uterine surgery, which puts you at greater risk for a uterine rupture. (The risks are higher, but the possibility of an induction is not entirely ruled out.)
- You're having placental problems, such as placenta previa (where the placenta covers all or part of the cervix) or heavy bleeding—you would be a candidate for a C-section.
- You have an active herpes lesion (you would need to have a Cesarean delivery to avoid passing the infection on to your baby).
- Your baby is not in a good position for birth (e.g., your baby is in a breech or transverse lie).

The Risks of Induction

Although induction can be a lifesaving tool, it's not without some risks. Some of these include:

- **Premature birth:** Your baby's gestational age may have been miscalculated, and her lungs, organs, and immune system may not be mature enough for her to thrive outside the womb.
- **Umbilical cord problems:** If your health care provider artificially ruptures your membranes to help induce labor, there's an increased risk that the umbilical cord could slip through the cervix before the baby (umbilical cord prolapse), which could put pressure on the umbilical cord, potentially decreasing the baby's oxygen supply. Umbilical cord prolapse is cause for an emergency C-section.
- **Uterine rupture:** If you've had a prior uterine surgery or C-section, you're at a slightly increased risk for uterine rupture along the scar tissue from your previous surgery.
- **Hemorrhage:** Induction increases the risk that your uterine muscles won't contract properly after delivery, resulting in excessive bleeding.
- **Increased odds for further interventions:** Studies have shown that having an induction can increase the odds that your baby would need to be delivered using forceps, vacuum extraction, or Cesarean delivery.

WHAT HAPPENS DURING AN INDUCTION?

When a woman gets induced, her cervix and uterus receive some type of natural, chemical, or medical influence intended to start labor. There are many ways to go about this, both inside and outside the hospital. Some work better than others, and there's room for debate over which methods are really effective and which are coincidentally effective (meaning labor started after using a technique, but it may have started anyway, without it). The following is a list of induction techniques that tend to be used at home or in birth centers:

Nipple stimulation causes a natural release of oxytocin that often leads to uterine contractions. During most stages of pregnancy, nipple stimulation during sex, bathing, or nursing an older baby won't cause strong enough contractions to stimulate labor. With an at-term pregnancy, however, when the cervix is already favorable for labor, it might be effective in starting labor for some women.

How do you do it? Use a breast pump, your partner, or your own hands to massage, roll, and/or suck the nipple for five minutes. Wait fifteen minutes and see whether there's any effect before trying again. You may have to repeat this cycle many times to keep contractions going. If labor doesn't take off on its own after a while, that's a sign you're not quite ready to deliver.

Does it work? An analysis of six medical trials (Kavanagh, et.al.) compared results of breast stimulation with no intervention and found a significant reduction in the number of women (62.7 percent versus 93.6 percent) not in labor within seventy-two hours. This success rate may be partly because partners often have sex after nipple stimulation.

Sex, specifically vaginal intercourse that results in the man ejaculating inside the vagina, may cause a release of prostaglandin hormones that stimulate labor. Cervical mucus also contains prostaglandins, and stimulation of the cervix may cause it to release labor-inducing hormones.

Does it work? Millions of women and centuries of experience say that sex may get labor started within hours to days after intercourse. Research published in the journal *Obstetrics and Gynecology* supports this claim and says that having frequent sex close to your due date can reduce the need for induction of labor. Another study, however, says sex doesn't work and, in fact, may actually delay labor. One more study says sex alone may not cause labor to start, but nipple stimulation during sex might. In low-risk women, however, there are no significant risks to giving it a try (and it makes most fathers/partners feel happy and useful). Please keep in mind that both nipple stimulation (by a partner) and sex should be used only at home, not in the hospital. Your labor nurses and health care providers have probably "seen it all," but witnessing sexual behavior should not be part of their job description. As with all sexual behavior, privacy and respect for all involved is important.

Acupuncture involves the use of small, sterile needles placed on several distinct points on the body by a trained professional to stimulate flow of energy (chi). In traditional Western medicine, acupuncture is thought to stimulate release of prostaglandins and oxytocin. There aren't enough studies on acupuncture success rates, but many women, acupuncturists, and cultures stand behind the claim that acupuncture is effective in getting labor started.

Castor oil and **enemas** are sometimes used to irritate the bowel and encourage it to empty its contents, which, in turn, may stimulate the uterus to do the same. There's a lot of anecdotal evidence that these methods are effective for some women whose cervices are very ready, but there are no substantial studies to prove it. Enemas might be more preferable than castor oil because castor oil has a very unpleasant taste and often causes nausea, vomiting, and diarrhea, sometimes for days after drinking it and often throughout the resulting labor.

Herbal supplements include those most commonly recommended by midwives—evening primrose oil, black cohosh, and red raspberry leaves. Sometimes used in combinations, these herbs might work as cervical ripening agents and to stimulate contractions. No clinical studies could be found to support their effectiveness for starting labor, though many midwives and women report they are both safe and effective.

One problem with herbal remedies is a lack of consistency in how they're dispensed and formulated, including recommendations for how to use them. The American Pregnancy Association and the Natural Medicines Database say black cohosh is considered likely unsafe (especially if the baby is preterm) during pregnancy. Raspberry leaf is considered likely safe during pregnancy. Primrose is considered possibly unsafe. The American Academy of Family Physicians says, "The risks and benefits of these agents are still unknown because the quality of evidence is based on a long tradition of use by a certain population and anecdotal case reports."

Before Your Induction

Unlike alternative techniques, there are many studies that support evidence on the risks, benefits, and effectiveness of inducing labor using traditional Western medical cervical ripening agents, artificial rupture of membranes, and Pitocin.

The success of any induction is based in large part on whether mother and baby are ready for birth. That's why, before any induction, the patient's health care provider should be certain that mom's cervix is favorable (ready for labor) and baby is mature enough for birth. That's evaluated with a Bishop score and accurate documentation of fetal age.

A Bishop score is a system used to determine whether the cervix is ready for induction based on cervical dilation, effacement, station, consistency, and position. Each criterion is given a score of 0 to 3 points. A Bishop score greater than 6 is considered appropriate for induction of labor, though many health care providers (including some hospitals) won't do elective inductions if the Bishop score is lower than 10 for first-time mothers and 8 for subsequent deliveries.

A favorable cervix. What does this feel like? It's soft, not firm, thin not thick, beginning to open (not tightly closed), low in the birth canal, and near the front wall of the vagina. It's buttery, squishy, stretchy, and ready to dilate.

Accurate documentation of fetal age is key to preventing prematurity when inducing labor. After more than a decade of elective, early inductions that resulted in skyrocketing rates of premature deliveries and NICU admissions, many hospitals are now banning any elective inductions (for nonmedical reasons) before 39 weeks. ACOG guidelines mandate that fetal age be well established by:

- A definite date for the first day of the last menstrual period
- An ultrasound measurement prior to 20 weeks gestation that supports gestational age of 39 weeks or greater
- Thirty-six weeks or longer since a positive blood or urine pregnancy test result
- Amniocentesis verifying fetal lung maturity
- Fetal heart tones documented as present for 30 weeks

Even with meeting one or more of these criteria, many babies need 39 weeks or longer to complete fetal development, and ultrasounds and dates for last menstrual period can be inaccurate. There's even a risk for prematurity when baby is born at 39 weeks. Even when amniocentesis (which is rarely done purely for preinduction reasons) determines that baby's lungs are mature, studies now indicate that important neurological development takes place in the last days to weeks of pregnancy.

Be sure you have a solid medical reason for why you need to be induced before you inadvertently short-change your baby's time in the uterus. If the reason outweighs the risks for induction, then by all means proceed. If your reason for induction is for convenience, scheduling, or minor discomfort, however, think twice. Though some hospitals ban all elective inductions, certain patients can still opt for one under certain conditions, such as those cited above. If you and your provider are considering an elective induction for nonmedical reasons (they can and do happen successfully for many patients who have good reasons to schedule their delivery), be prepared to consider all the risks and benefits outlined by your provider. Then be prepared to take a calculated risk that your induction will go smoothly. Chances are good that if you're at term, your cervix is favorable, and your Bishop score is appropriate, your induction can result in a healthy vaginal delivery for both mom and baby.

During Your Induction

Every induction starts with admission to the hospital. You'll be escorted to your labor room, change

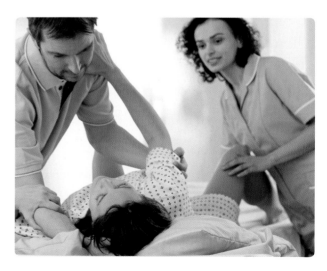

Your cervix will most likely be examined before your induction to determine whether it is ready to dilate. While most women aren't crazy about vaginal/cervical exams, they shouldn't be terribly uncomfortable and should be brief.

your clothes, sign paperwork, and begin fetal heart monitoring. Your vital signs will be checked and an IV will be started (usually in your wrist, hand, or arm). A blood test may be sent to the lab.

Your cervix will probably be examined and your Bishop score determined. After an initial interpretation of your fetal heart and contraction patterns, your health care provider will decide how to proceed with your induction. That may mean use of cervical ripening agents, artificial rupture of membranes, or going straight to Pitocin.

Some cervical ripening techniques, including prostaglandin gel, balloons, and stripping of membranes, are performed on an outpatient basis in some birth centers and hospitals. In other facilities, balloons and prostaglandin products are only used on an inpatient basis.

How Cervical Ripening Works

Cervical ripening agents help get your cervix ready for labor. It's no easy job. Before it can dilate, your cervix needs to do a complete about-face. After nine months of staying solidly closed and keeping everything safely inside the uterus, it now has to soften, thin, stretch, and get into a good position, so it can dilate and let your baby out. This process can take

Inside Information

Very often, inductions are a two- or even three-day event. They often start with cervical ripening, to get the cervix ready to dilate. This can take several hours or all day and is often done as an overnight procedure. This is usually followed by IV Pitocin administration. If a full day of Pitocin doesn't do the job (and if amniotic membranes are still intact), and the cervix isn't dilated very far, many doctors and midwives will turn off the Pitocin, shut everything down for the night, and start again the next day.

Sometimes, if the cervix isn't ready to budge, they'll shut everything down for much longer (perhaps a week) and send the patient home. As long as mom and baby are well enough to continue the pregnancy, this is often a safer way to proceed than to push an induction that's going nowhere. Continuing an induction that isn't working generally leads to a C-section.

Because you don't know how long it will take for active labor to kick in or to deliver your baby, think carefully about when to call your family and friends to wait at the hospital. Inductions frequently take a lot longer than spontaneous labor, especially if you need cervical ripening or more than one day of Pitocin. If your fan club is at the hospital waiting for your baby right from the start, they're going to wait a very long time. That can make you feel like you're "on the clock" and under pressure to perform. It's often a better plan to wait until labor is well on its way and delivery is within a couple hours before calling anyone to come to the hospital other than your essential labor support team.

hours, days, and even weeks (and happens naturally during the last stages of pregnancy) or can be done overnight at the hospital. Inductions that are done with an unfavorable cervix have a higher failure rate, which may lead to complications such as prolonged labor, infection, maternal fatigue, fetal intolerance to labor, and C-section. These are the devices and medications used for cervical ripening:

Mechanical dilators work by putting pressure on the cervix to release prostaglandins. They're usually left in place for six or more hours and very often, overnight. They include:

- Natural or synthetic hygroscopic dilators (Laminaria japonicum or Lamicel). These aren't commonly used in most health care facilities anymore because they're associated with a higher risk for infection than other techniques and products. They are inserted inside the cervix to absorb endocervical and local tissue fluids. This causes the dilators to expand and provide controlled mechanical pressure. These devices can sometimes be used on an outpatient basis, which means the patient can have them inserted at her health care provider's office or in the hospital. Then she can go home to rest while they do their job.

- Balloon devices such as a Foley catheter (usually used to drain urine from the bladder) or a device specifically designed for use inside the cervix and/or uterus are usually used on an inpatient basis. Some birth centers and hospitals may provide the option of letting mom go home overnight after having the balloon placed. The catheter is inserted into the cervix. A balloon in the tip of the cervix is then filled with water (through a syringe attached to the catheter end that's outside the vagina) until it stays in place to provide continuous cervical pressure.

Procedures: Don't let the word *procedures* scare you. These techniques (which include stripping or artificially rupturing the membrane) to stimulate cervical ripening and contractions don't require a trip to the operating room.

- Stripping the membranes is among the gentlest methods for stimulating the cervix to ripen on its own. Your health care provider will insert her finger into the cervical opening and rotate it around the inside to detach the amniotic membrane from inside the cervix. This stimulates prostaglandin production and might cause cramping and spotting. This is often done in the midwife or doctor's office; afterward patients go home and wait for labor to start.

- Artificial rupture of membranes (a.k.a. *amniotomy*) by itself used to be a common technique for inducing labor but isn't currently popular because it hasn't been proven to be as effective as other techniques. It can work very well for some patients who are dilated 5 centimeters or more without the use of other induction interventions. (It is often used in conjunction with medication, though.) Your health care provider will use a long plastic hook (it looks like a flat crochet hook) to snag the amniotic membranes and break them. The exam might be uncomfortable, but breaking the membranes doesn't hurt.

The release of fluid combined with pressure from the baby's head being applied to the cervix usually starts contractions within several hours to a couple of days. Once the membranes are ruptured, however, there's no turning back, and baby must be delivered within a day or so. Here's what ACOG says:

> "Artificial rupture of the membranes may be a method of labor induction, especially if the condition of the cervix is favorable. Used alone for inducing labor, amniotomy can be associated with unpredictable and sometimes long intervals before the onset of contractions. There is insufficient evidence on the efficacy and safety of amniotomy alone for labor induction. In a trial of amniotomy combined with early oxytocin infusion compared with amniotomy alone, the induction-to-delivery interval was shorter with the amniotomy-plus-oxytocin method."

Pharmaceutical methods, which include prostaglandin gel and prostaglandin inserts, contain the same ingredients your own cervix provides to soften, thin, and prepare for labor.

- Prostaglandin gel (Prepidil) is squirted through a syringe into the area around the cervix and left in place for several hours or overnight. Application can be repeated every four hours up to three times. The patient and baby are monitored after gel is administered.
- Prostaglandin inserts (Cervidil) come in a thin, flat, rectangular tablet attached to a string. They're placed behind the cervix, left in place for up to twelve hours, and removed just like a tampon (by pulling the string). Many facilities will monitor the patient for two or more hours after insertion of Cervidil and, depending on circumstances, remove the monitor after that. Cervidil can cause strong uterine contractions in some patients, however, which might mean they need to remain on the monitors for a longer period of time or even continuously.
- Misoprostol (Cytotec) tablets are synthetic prostaglandin. Misoprostol is not officially labeled by the Food and Drug Administration for use as a cervical ripener but is among the most commonly used products for this purpose. It is also very effective for stopping postdelivery bleeding. Its official use is for the prevention and treatment of stomach ulcers. Misoprostol tablets are usually cut into quarters, and one tiny pill scrap is placed behind the cervix. It can also be administered orally, though most American practitioners use the intravaginal method. Misoprostol doses can be repeated every four hours. The patient has to lie down for at least thirty minutes after administration (to keep it from falling out) and must stay on continuous fetal monitoring for one to three hours before getting up.

Sometimes all it takes is one of these cervical ripening agents or techniques to get labor started. That can be a plus, because it may mean mom won't have to be tethered to a monitor or need an IV during labor. More often, however, these methods need to be followed by use of IV Pitocin.

Induction with IV Pitocin

Your IV will be attached to tubing (called the primary IV line) and a main IV bag filled with Lactated Ringer's or LR (a basic solution that contains no medications). In addition, you'll have a separate IV bag filled with LR plus Pitocin. This will be attached to its own IV tubing, which will be threaded into a computerized IV pump and plugged into a port in your primary IV line (near the location where the IV is inserted into your arm).

Your nurse will program the Pitocin pump to start at a low initial dose (about 1 to 2 milliunits or MUs) and will increase it by 1 or 2 MUs every twenty to thirty minutes. Your contractions might take hours to start, or they might begin shortly after you start getting Pitocin. Your nurse will continue increasing the Pitocin dose using the IV pump until you're having regular contractions. She might have to increase or decrease the amount of Pitocin you receive periodically (called titrating the dose) so you continue having the right number of contractions.

What's the right number? Your nurse will monitor your contractions along with your baby's heart rate. The goal is for you to have between three and five contractions in ten minutes (averaged over a thirty-minute period) that are strong enough to cause cervical change. Occasionally the Pitocin infusion can be turned off entirely if labor is progressing quickly.

If there are more than five contractions in ten minutes, that's called *tachysystole*, which could cause fetal distress and/or damage to the uterus. If you have too many contractions, your nurse will dial down the amount of Pitocin or stop the infusion for a while. This is usually enough to space out contractions. After a short period of time, the Pitocin will be restarted at a lower dose.

Your nurse can increase the pump to deliver up to 20 MUs of Pitocin. Sometimes a dose higher than 20 MUs is needed, but the health care provider often must provide special orders to give more. The highest dose allowed is 40 MUs, but it's unusual that more than 20 MUs are ever needed.

There's no way to determine in advance how much Pitocin a patient will need. It's individualized and depends on how many Pitocin receptors are available in her body and how ready her body is to be in labor. That's why careful monitoring and custom titrating of the dose is required.

How Induction Changes Fetal Heart Monitoring

In many hospitals, induction is accompanied by constant fetal monitoring. That means that once the contraction and fetal heart monitor belts are on, they'll stay on until after delivery. This reduces mom's ability to walk, take a bath or shower, use the birthing ball, or change positions during labor. It's not impossible, just more challenging. In many hospitals, however, once a stable dose of Pitocin has been reached and safe fetal heart and contraction patterns have been established, the patient can be monitored intermittently. That means the belts can come off for about twenty minutes out of every hour (unless the Pitocin dose needs to be increased) so mom can move around.

Many hospitals and birth centers now have wireless fetal heart monitoring (called telemetry). Telemetry can be great for walking and bouncing on the ball. With certain telemetry units that are compatible with water, mom can even get into the tub. It can be challenging to keep track of the heartbeat, which might be annoying for mom and her providers, but the added mobility telemetry allows makes it worth the extra effort.

Pitocin and frequent contractions can cause mom's blood pressure to change, so her nurse will check her blood pressure, pulse, respirations, and possibly her temperature more frequently. Her blood pressure and pulse will be assessed every time her Pitocin dose changes and every hour to two hours throughout labor. If her amniotic membranes are ruptured, her temperature will be checked every hour or two.

Q: *How long will induction take?*
A: That depends. For some women (usually those with second or subsequent pregnancies), it only takes a number of hours for Pitocin to move a labor through to delivery. For other women (first time mothers or those whose body wasn't ready for labor), it can take a day or two and even longer.

Q: *What if induction doesn't work?*
A: Sometimes inductions don't work. Cervical ripeners and Pitocin can almost always cause contractions, but that doesn't mean they'll cause cervical change. This is especially common for first-time mothers or those who aren't close to their due date. When that happens, sometimes the best course of action is to turn off the Pitocin and monitor for a while to make sure contractions are subsiding and baby is stable and

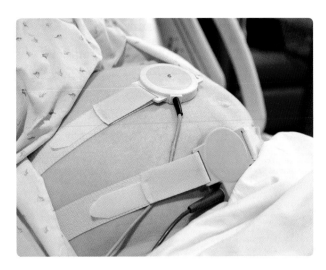

Induction is typically accompanied by close fetal monitoring to determine contraction frequency and length and to evaluate how your baby is tolerating labor. You may still be able to walk and move around, change positions, and take a break from the monitor.

- Let mom go home and wait for spontaneous labor *or*
- Let mom go home and try and induce another day *or*
- Let mom sleep in the hospital overnight and start Pitocin again the next day *or*
- Re-administer cervical ripening agents and either send mom home or restart Pitocin the next day.

The key to being able to do an induction over a couple (or a few) days is to leave the amniotic membranes intact. Once they've been ruptured, there's increased risk for infection and increased pressure to get mom delivered sooner than later, even if that means a C-section.

Sometimes even a couple days of induction won't do the trick. If it's very important that the baby be delivered, the only other option is a C-section.

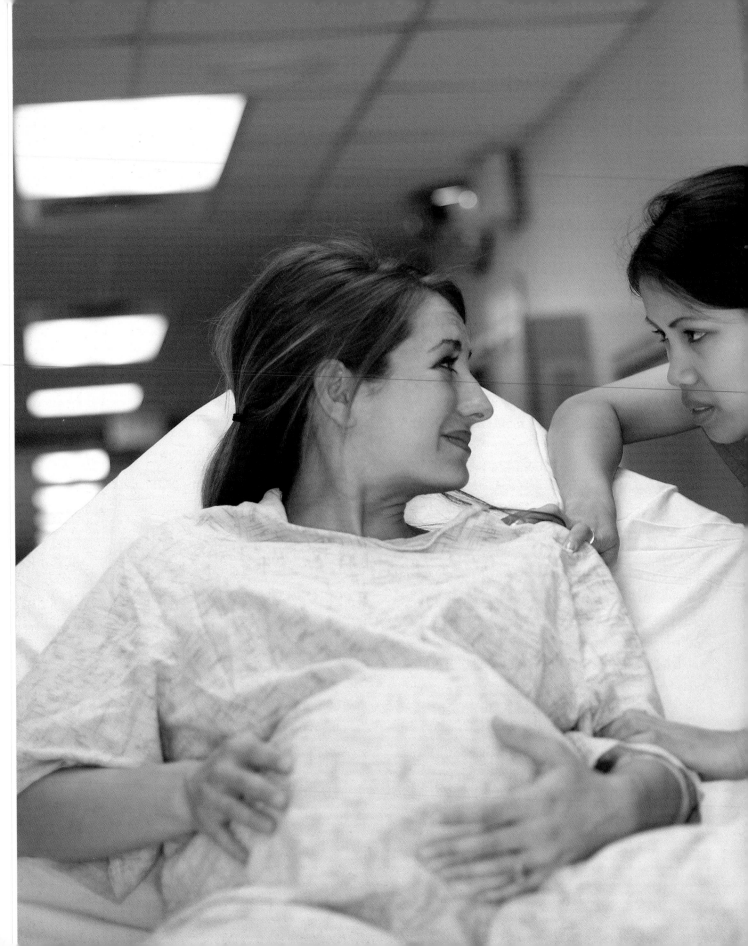

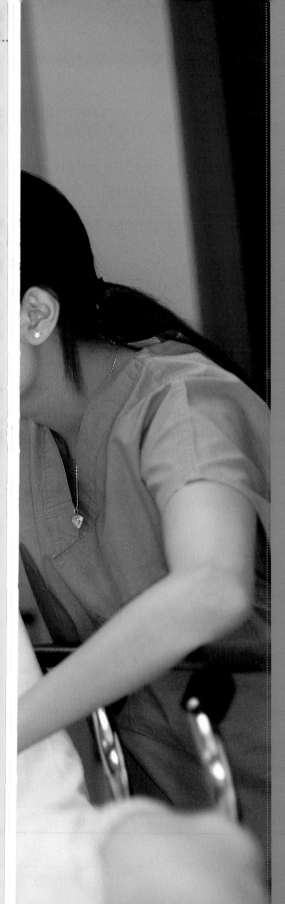

CHAPTER 7

Vaginal Birth after Cesarean (VBAC)

What it is, why it may or may not be right for you, pros and cons, and how to prepare for this labor path

Vaginal birth after Cesarean (a.k.a. VBAC, pronounced *vee-bak*) means a woman has had a C-section and then has a vaginal delivery with a subsequent baby.

She goes through what's called a trial of labor after Cesarean (TOLAC), so called because the woman and her doctor hope that whatever events were responsible for her first C-section won't be a problem for her next labor. In other words, they're giving vaginal birth a try (a "trial"), hoping for a safe delivery, and in most cases are successful.

Although a VBAC is not recommended for some women, most make excellent candidates. The American Congress of Obstetricians and Gynecologists (ACOG) predict that about 70 percent of women who undergo a TOLAC will successfully have a VBAC and deliver a healthy baby.

On the surface, VBAC seems fairly straightforward, but in reality it has become one of the most controversial issues women and their providers face when it comes to childbirth.

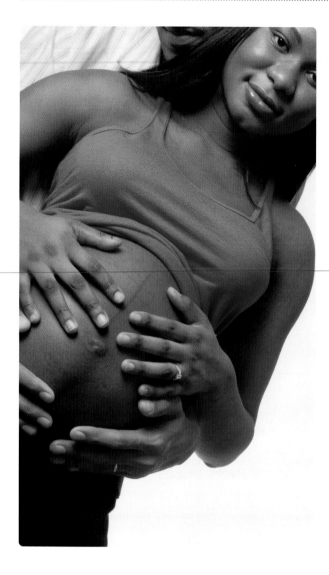

The risks associated with having a trial of labor after Cesarean delivery, and/or a VBAC, include:

- Uterine rupture
- Maternal hemorrhage
- Infection
- Operative injury
- Thromboembolism (a clot that breaks loose and travels to other areas of the body)
- Hysterectomy
- Death

Note that many of these are inherent risks in any type of delivery, but women who attempt a TOLAC should be counseled about them.

What if you're carrying multiples? Studies have shown that women who are carrying twins who attempt VBAC have similar outcomes to women carrying single babies who attempt VBAC.

HOW TO PREPARE FOR A VBAC

Want to increase the odds you'll have a successful VBAC? Start with the following:

- Choose a health care provider who supports VBAC. One of the most important things you can do to prepare for a VBAC birth is to find a provider who supports them, in theory and practice. Ask to see your health care provider's VBAC success rates—look for someone who has a good track record of successful VBACs and a lower-than-average rate of Cesarean deliveries. (In general, C-section rates are about 30 percent, while successful VBAC rates are about 70 percent.)

with a classical or T-incision, prior uterine rupture, or extensive uterine surgery), are not generally considered to be candidates.

In 2010, ACOG also recommended that women who've had two prior Cesarean deliveries should be counseled about VBAC and offered a TOLAC if they don't present other risk factors.

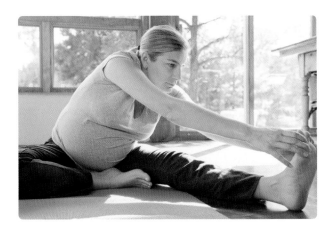

One of the best determinants for having a healthy vaginal delivery is to have a healthy mother with a normal body weight. Exercise during your pregnancy to feel strong and healthy during labor and increase chances for a successful TOLAC.

- Consider hiring a doula. Working with a doula, or other support person who's knowledgeable about natural childbirth, can increase the likelihood that you'll have a successful labor and birth.

- Educate yourself about VBAC. Read as much as you can about VBAC, including birth stories of women who've gone through their own TOLAC.

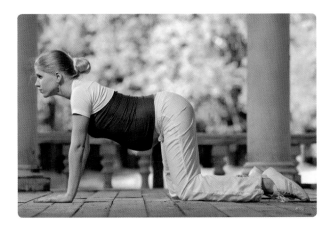

Practice labor positions such as this hands-and-knees (all-fours) position to open up the pelvic region and ease baby through the birth canal.

Consider taking a childbirth education class that focuses specifically on VBAC. For instance, many doulas, midwives, or local Lamaze chapters offer private VBAC classes.

- Focus on nutrition and exercise. With your health care provider's approval, be sure to exercise regularly and focus on good nutrition. If you're feeling strong and healthy when you go into labor, you'll be more likely to have a successful TOLAC.

- Practice labor positions. Before you go into labor, practice some of the labor positions—such as squats, lunges, or getting down on all fours—that have been shown to open up the pelvic region and ease the baby through the birth canal, thereby increasing your odds of having a vaginal delivery. (See chapter 10 for more on labor positions.)

What's Different about VBAC Labor, Delivery, and Postpartum Care

Other than those items listed below, there are little other differences in the delivery of your baby or placenta, or the postpartum care that you'll receive. And yes—you can still have that epidural!

- **Where you'll give birth:** ACOG recommends that you labor and deliver at a facility capable of emergency deliveries because of the risks associated with TOLAC, and because uterine rupture and other complications can come on suddenly and unpredictably. However, ACOG's position has been a matter of great discussion. Many members of the medical community

Inside Information

Many hospitals and doctors refuse to "allow" their patients to have a VBAC, even though ACOG, the American College of Nurse Midwives, and the World Health Organization agree that it's a safe option for most women. Why the objection? In the approximately 1 percent of VBACs that result in uterine rupture, the chance for maternal or newborn death and a subsequent lawsuit is greater than with a routine C-section or vaginal birth. Even though uterine rupture is a rare complication that does not usually result in death, many insurance companies refuse to cover hospitals and doctors who allow VBACs. No insurance means that hospitals and doctors simply won't do them.

Though ACOG guidelines state that TOLAC and VBAC can be safe and should be encouraged, they also state that "TOLAC be undertaken in facilities with staff immediately available to provide emergency care" if anything goes wrong. That is generally interpreted to mean the OB and anesthetist have to be in the building for the entire labor and delivery. That sounds good on paper, but in reality, that's not the way our health care system operates in many parts of the country. Most doctors can't hang out on the labor unit throughout a patient's entire labor. They have patients to see in their offices and dinner to have with their spouses and children. In addition, many hospitals can't employ a full-time, on-site anesthetist/anesthesiologist available twenty-four hours per day. Instead, they call them in from home or their offices, with the expectation they'll be on the labor unit within about twenty minutes.

That's why, when doctors and hospitals tallied up the risks associated with VBAC, the superhigh insurance rates, and the new physician availability expectations, virtually all doctors and hospitals slammed the doors shut on VBAC.

But that's not the only reason why many doctors are reluctant to participate in VBACs. There's also the fear factor. Though most doctors will never experience having a patient hemorrhage and die from uterine rupture, all doctors, midwives, and nurses have seen mothers and babies with bad outcomes for a variety of reasons. These are frightening tragedies that impact health care providers on a deep, personal, emotional level that sticks with them forever. Very few providers walk away from a traumatic patient event unchanged. They grieve and feel personally responsible, even if, in reality, they did not cause the incident; it simply happened on their watch. It changes the way they think about their work, skills, and practice. It also makes them want to avoid risk, both consciously and unconsciously.

In addition, health care professionals go under the microscope as supervisors, legal teams, and risk assessment personnel grill them about what happened and how they were involved. It's an anxiety-provoking situation that no provider wants to go through. Many health care providers decide they won't put their heads, hearts, and practices at risk for this kind of anxiety and tragedy, even if the chances are extremely slim that it would ever happen to them.

Patient care is a two-way relationship, and though all pregnant women are at risk for unexpected complications, so are their health care providers. VBACs have provided an excellent opportunity for the obstetric community to examine this relationship and evolve to meet its challenges.

would like to increase availability of VBAC in hospital-based birth centers and rural and community hospitals.

- **Monitoring:** Most hospitals and health care providers require continuous electronic fetal monitoring for a TOLAC. Your nurse or health care provider will watch you closely for any signs that have been associated with uterine rupture, such as fetal bradycardia (an abnormally slow fetal heart rate), increased uterine contractions, vaginal bleeding, loss of fetal station (station is a sign of how "engaged" the baby's head is in the pelvis), or a sudden onset of intense uterine pain.

- **Drugs for labor induction or augmentation:** According to the ACNM, induction of labor should only be undertaken when the benefits outweigh the risks and only in the hospital setting following consultation with a physician who is available to perform a Cesarean.

Although induction of labor may remain an option for certain women having a TOLAC, you may not be able to have your labor augmented with Pitocin. Some studies have shown an association between labor augmentation with Pitocin and uterine rupture, while others have shown no correlation. (You *can* still be induced with Pitocin. There is a small increase in the risk of uterine rupture, but ACOG states that Pitocin is an option as long as the risk is discussed with the patient. For Pitocin augmentation, the risk is not as clear. It is also not clear whether more Pitocin is associated with more uterine ruptures, and how much is too much.)

Misoprostol should not be used for cervical ripening or labor induction, as it has been shown to increase the rate of uterine rupture. Data on prostaglandin use for cervical ripening is not as clear, but is generally not done either. ACOG says that given the lack of compelling data suggesting an increased risk with mechanical dilation and cervical catheters, these can still be an option for TOLAC candidates who have an unfavorable cervix. The bottom line is that when you start with an unfavorable cervix and/or need to be induced, your chances of having a successful VBAC are lower, so you need to consider the risks and benefits of using medications or devices to induce labor and decide with your provider what the best and safest choice is for you.

Patient care is a two-way relationship, and though all pregnant women are at risk for unexpected complications, so are their health care providers.

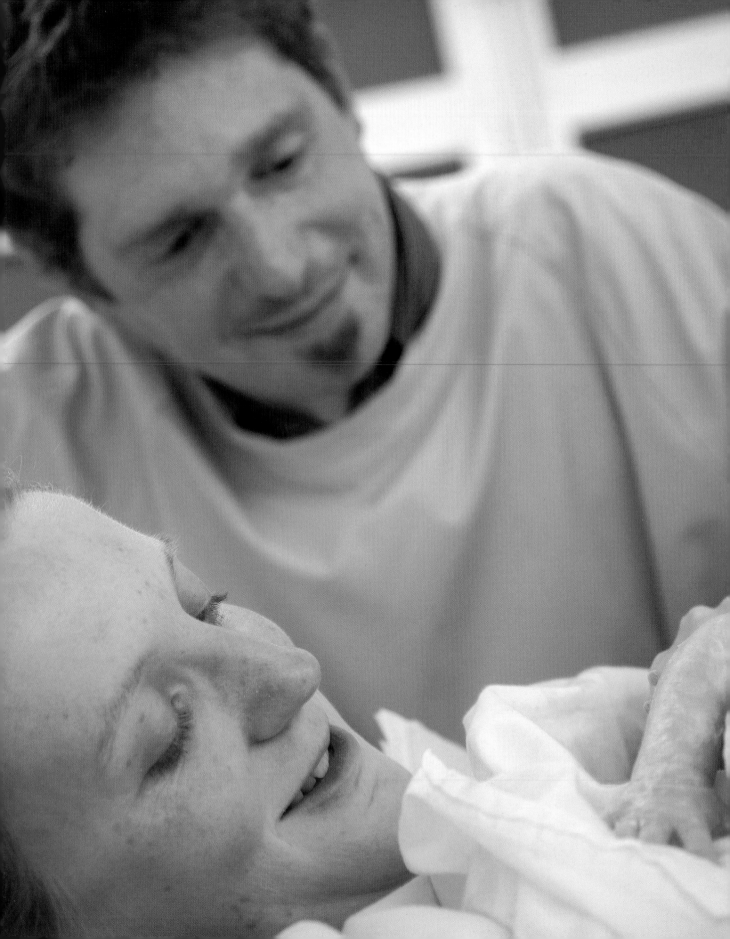

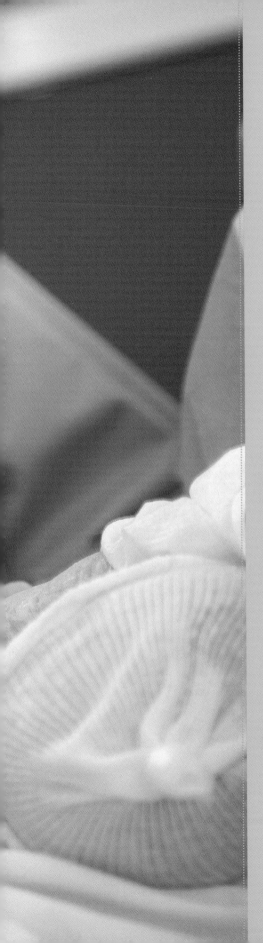

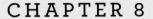
Planned Cesarean Birth in a Hospital

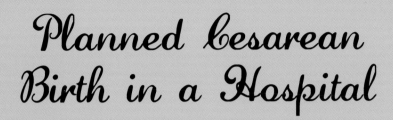

What it is, why it may or may not be right for you, pros and cons, and how to prepare for this labor path

There are certain situations where a vaginal delivery is simply not the best course of action for mom or baby, and your health care provider may want to plan for a Cesarean section, where the baby will be delivered through incisions in the mother's abdomen and uterus. (In the next chapter, we'll talk about unplanned Cesarean deliveries.) Circumstances that may call for a planned Cesarean delivery include:

- Mom is carrying multiples (sometimes mom can deliver vaginally, but not always).
- The baby is in a breech position (where the feet would enter the birth canal first) or a transverse position (lying sideways across the uterus) instead of a head-down position.
- There's a complication with the placenta, such as placenta previa (where the placenta covers all or part of the cervix).
- Mom has an active case of herpes, HIV, or other infection, where a vaginal delivery would risk infecting the baby.
- Mom has had previous C-sections or uterine surgery and is not a candidate for a vaginal birth after Cesarean (VBAC). (See chapter 7 for more on VBAC.)
- Mom has a serious medical condition, such as heart disease.

- The baby has certain birth defects, such as severe spina bifida, where it may not be safe for the baby to go through the birth canal. (In the case of spina bifida, the baby's exposed neural tissue could be injured.)

In some instances, mom may request a Cesarean delivery for nonmedical reasons. These deliveries are called Cesarean delivery upon maternal request. We'll talk more about those below.

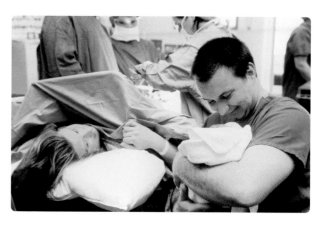

Planned C-sections can be beautiful deliveries, especially if your hospital has family-friendly policies. Your partner can usually be by your side, and if everyone is stable, your baby can stay with you.

PROS AND CONS OF A PLANNED CESAREAN DELIVERY

Pros

- For some women with the complications listed above, a C-section is considered safer than a vaginal delivery, and in many cases (such as with placenta previa), a C-section can be a lifesaving procedure.

- A planned Cesarean often takes place in a more controlled atmosphere, as compared to spontaneous labor or an emergency C-section.

- A planned Cesarean allows the parents and health care providers to know exactly when the baby will be born, which can be helpful when planning for dad to be at the delivery and for planning a work leave, care for other children and dependents, and the availability of labor support people.

- A planned Cesarean can help a woman ensure that her own obstetrician will deliver her baby.

Cons

- A C-section is a major abdominal surgery, which poses certain risks for mom such as infection, blood loss, blood clots, injury to the bowel or bladder, and reactions to the drugs or anesthesia used.

- Your body will need more time to recover from a C-section than from a vaginal delivery. Expect to be in the hospital for three to four days after delivery (as opposed to two days with a vaginal delivery), and it can take up to six weeks or more to fully recover from the surgery.

- It can be difficult to pinpoint the exact gestational age of the baby, which means that there's a greater risk that some babies may be delivered before their lungs or immune system are fully mature. (However, because many women now get first-trimester ultrasounds, the reality is that the dating is usually pretty good.)

- C-sections typically cost more than vaginal deliveries. (In 2003, the average charges associated with uncomplicated C-sections were $11,500, which is more than $5,000 greater than the mean charge for all routine vaginal deliveries.)

- Some women may have some initial trouble breastfeeding their babies after a Cesarean delivery, as they may have trouble sitting up or getting into a comfortable position to feed the baby because of pain from the surgery.

- Some women feel disappointed by the experience of a Cesarean birth, because they don't feel like active participants in the process, and rather that their deliveries happened to them.

- Having one C-section may necessitate C-sections for subsequent pregnancies (see chapter 7 on VBAC for more information).

- Babies born via C-section are more likely to have breathing problems than babies born vaginally. Some attribute this to the fact that as babies travel through the birth canal, the pressure of the uterine muscles on the baby's body helps to squeeze mucus and other fluids out of the baby's airway naturally.

- Having a C-section puts you at an increased risk for certain complications in subsequent pregnancies, such as placenta previa, placenta accreta, and placental abruption.

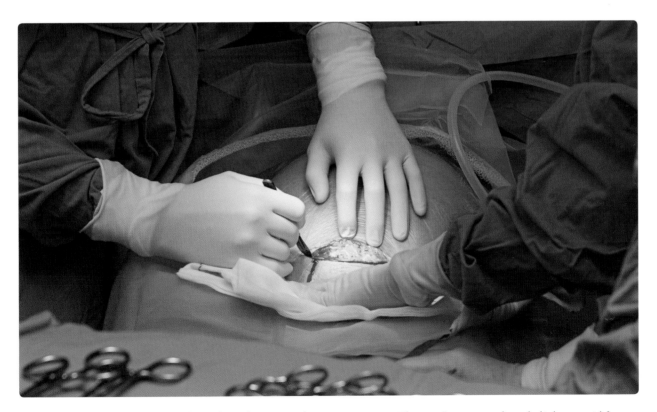

Your uterine scar can increase risks for placental complications in subsequent pregnancies. The more C-sections you have, the higher your risk for placenta previa, placenta accreta, and placental abruption.

When a C-Section Is Requested, Not Required

Some women may request a Cesarean birth even if vaginal delivery is an option. This decision should be weighed carefully and discussed with your health care provider. As with any surgery, there are risks and complications to consider. Your hospital stay will be longer than with a vaginal birth. Also, the more Cesarean births a woman has, the greater her risk for complications and problems with future pregnancies. Therefore, an elective Cesarean section is not recommended for women who wish to have many children.

The American Congress of Obstetricians and Gynecologists (ACOG) defines *Cesarean delivery on maternal request* as "a primary Cesarean delivery at the request of the mother, in the absence of any medical or obstetric indication." According to

Inside Information

Ask any woman who's had an unplanned or emergency C-section and then a planned one with a subsequent pregnancy, and she'll tell you that by comparison, planned C-sections are a piece of cake. Sure, there might be some presurgery jitters, but in general, they're much easier and less stressful because parents know what to expect and haven't already been exhausted by a long, challenging labor. There's less anxiety because baby isn't in distress and mom isn't in labor. They're calm, organized, and quick.

In fact, planned C-sections can be very beautiful deliveries. They're still major surgery, but if your hospital has family-friendly policies that make bonding, rooming in, breastfeeding, and family time a priority, then a C-section birth can be just as miraculous and special as a vaginal birth.

As soon as you know you're having a C-section, contact the maternity unit at your hospital and find out about their policies for keeping mother and baby together, breastfeeding, and rooming in. If they don't have a family-friendly plan already nailed down, then it's time to negotiate for what you want. Ask your health care provider to support you.

As long as you and your baby don't require any out-of-the-ordinary medical care, and as long as someone in your family (or a doula) can stay with you to help with baby care, there's no reason why you and your baby shouldn't be together, just like you would be with a vaginal birth. If you do feel lousy after surgery, however, don't beat yourself up about not spending every moment with your baby. You just had major surgery and you need to recover. (See "The Real Deal" in this chapter.)

If your hospital has lactation specialists, ask for a consultation as soon as possible after surgery. Complications from C-sections sometimes interfere with breastfeeding.

ACOG, a potential benefit of Cesarean delivery on maternal request is a decreased risk of hemorrhage for the mother, while potential risks include a longer maternal hospital stay, an increased risk of respiratory problems for the baby, and greater complications in subsequent pregnancies, including uterine rupture and placental implantation.

ACOG says that Cesarean delivery on maternal request should not be performed before the gestational age of 39 weeks has been accurately determined, unless there is documentation of lung maturity. The organization also says that Cesarean delivery on maternal request is not recommended for women who would like to have several children, given that the risks of placenta previa, placenta accreta, and the need for a hysterectomy at the time of delivery increase with each Cesarean delivery.

... in general, [planned C-sections are] much easier and less stressful because parents know what to expect and haven't already been exhausted by a long, challenging labor.

Statistics and Controversy Surrounding Planned Cesarean Deliveries

Approximately one in three babies in the United States is currently delivered via C-section, according to a data brief from the National Center for Health Statistics (NCHS). Key findings from the report say that:

- The Cesarean rate rose by 53 percent from 1996 to 2007, reaching 32 percent—the highest rate ever reported in the United States.
- Cesarean rates also increased for infants at all gestational ages; from 1996 to 2006, preterm infants had the highest rates.

How Does the U.S. C-Section Rate Compare with Other Countries?

Here's how the U.S. C-section rate compares with some other countries, according to a report from the World Health Organization for 2008:

COUNTRY	CESAREAN SECTION RATE
Brazil	45.9 percent
Iran	41.9 percent
Mexico	37.8 percent
Italy	38.2 percent
Australia	30.3 percent
U.S.	30.3 percent
Canada	26.3 percent
U.K.	22.0 percent
France	18.8 percent
Japan	17.4 percent
Sweden	17.3 percent
Uganda	3.1 percent

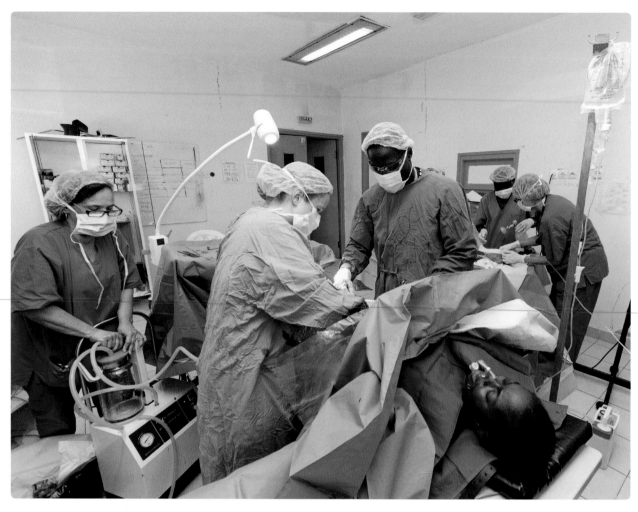

The World Health Organization says the most appropriate C-section rate to keep mothers and babies safe is between 5 and 15 percent. Pictured: A woman undergoing a C-section in an African hospital.

Why the high C-section rates? The NCHS study says that "in addition to clinical reasons, nonmedical factors suggested for the . . . rise of the Cesarean rate may include maternal demographic characteristics (e.g., older maternal age), physician practice patterns, maternal choice, more conservative practice guidelines, and legal pressures."

In many cases, the benefits of C-section far outnumber the risks. C-section can be a lifesaving tool when mom's or baby's health or lives are at risk. However, critics argue that it's not plausible that one in three women is unable to safely deliver her baby vaginally; that the rise in C-section rates does not correspond to a rise in healthy outcomes for moms and babies; that C-sections land moms and babies back in the hospital or intensive care units more often than vaginal deliveries; and that too many C-sections are doing more harm than good. However, physicians cite reasons such as an increasingly older, more obese and unhealthy population of women giving birth for a rise in complications during pregnancy and labor, as well as an increase in the number of women delivering multiples because of fertility treatments. And, in a climate where you're currently more likely to have a C-section in a subsequent pregnancy if you had a C-section for your first delivery, it's no wonder that C-section rates have skyrocketed.

However, recent data shows that the rising C-section trend may be on the way out. The Cesarean delivery rate declined slightly to 32.8 percent (from 32.9 percent)—the first drop in the rate in more than a decade, according to a 2010 report from the U.S. Department of Health and Human Services' National Vital Statistics System. Time will tell whether this slight dip will continue toward a more solid downward trend.

WHAT HAPPENS IN THE HOSPITAL PRIOR TO A PLANNED C-SECTION?

A planned C-section can arguably be among the calmest, smoothest, most expedient ways to have a baby. You know how and (give or take a few minutes) when your baby will be born. There's very little pain involved in the birthing process (though there is quite a lot more after surgery), and the whole operation takes little time (though there is more recovery time involved than with a vaginal birth). Here's what happens when you have a planned C-section.

On the day you and your doctor decide is your baby's birthday, you'll check into the maternity unit of your hospital. Your check-in time will be two to three hours before your scheduled C-section. For example, if your C-section is planned for 7:30 a.m., you'll be expected at the hospital by 5:30 a.m. or earlier. A lot of C-sections are planned for early in the morning because it means your doctor can do your surgery before office hours.

After being greeted at the nurse's station, you'll be escorted to your room. It might be the room you'll return to after surgery or it might be a presurgical room.

You'll be given a hospital gown (put it on so the opening is in the back) and asked to get into bed. Patients sometimes ask to stay in their own clothing, but that's a bad idea. Surgery is messy, and we don't want to ruin your clothes. Hospital gowns are made of clean fabric that doesn't contain anything that could interfere with surgical instruments and solutions. They're easy to remove, in case we need to change you quickly. Don't worry about the fit. There are gowns in a variety of sizes to accommodate every body.

Once you're in bed, your nurse will assess how your baby is doing through fetal monitoring. She may or may not put on a contraction monitor. Most women are not in labor when they're admitted for a planned C-section, so evaluating contraction patterns isn't always necessary. Occasionally, however, a woman will already be in early or active labor on her surgery date. She might be given medication to make contractions stop or have her surgery time moved up a bit.

Your nurse will check your temperature, blood pressure, heart rate, respirations, and reflexes, and she'll document everything in your medical record on the computer. She'll ask about your health history, allergies, medications, surgical and anesthesia history, family history, and other questions.

One of the most important questions she'll ask is when was the last time you had anything to eat or drink. It's essential that your stomach be empty before surgery. You can't have surgery if you've had anything to eat or drink within eight hours because anesthesia and surgery sometimes make patients vomit, which could be inhaled into the lungs and cause pneumonia. Once your nurse is certain you haven't eaten, she and the doctor will have you sign paperwork giving consent to have a C-section.

A nurse will start your IV, probably in your wrist, forearm, hand, or (if there's no better site) the inside of your elbow. The elbow site isn't ideal

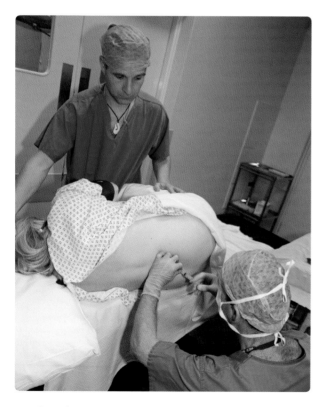

Spinal anesthesia is used in many planned C-sections and is administered in either a sitting or side-lying position. It starts to work quickly and ensures you won't feel pain during your surgery, though you might feel movement and pressure.

because you'll need your IV for several hours or days after surgery, and it can get in the way when you hold your baby. She'll hang a bag of Lactated Ringer's (a plain, nonmedicated IV solution) or other nonmedicated IV solution, run the first bag of fluid into your vein quickly, and hang a second bag. This main bag of IV fluid provides hydration throughout surgery and is used to administer a postdelivery dose of Pitocin and other medications. Just prior to surgery, you'll also receive IV antibiotics, given in a different IV bag plugged into a port on your IV line. After delivery, your IV line will be used for pain medication and other drugs you might need.

A side note about IVs: Labor and delivery units use big IV needles in case they need to give you blood during or after surgery. Red blood cells are large cells that must be transfused through a large needle so they won't break or tear. Also, they need to give you large quantities of fluids before (and sometimes during) surgery, and the larger the needle, the quicker they'll go into your vein.

Ask your nurse to numb your skin with a lidocaine or saline injection, a numbing ointment, or other anesthetic solution before she inserts the IV needle. What if she can't get the IV in on the first try? You might have challenging veins (small, slippery, or full of valves). Let her try a second time. If she still doesn't get it in, ask for another nurse, just in case it's her skills (and not your veins) that are the problem.

Your nurse or a lab technician will draw blood, and a sample will be held in the blood bank to verify your blood type in the rare event that you need a blood transfusion.

Your nurse will clip the hair in the area where your C-section incision will be located, just above your bikini line. Having a hair-free surgical site makes it easier for your surgeon to see where she's working, stitch the incision closed again, and remove your bandage later on.

Your doctor and anesthetist might come in to talk with you in your pre-op room before surgery, or you might not see them until you get to the operating room. You can probably walk to the operating room, accompanied by your husband/partner and your nurse, but if you're feeling nervous and wobbly, you can certainly request a wheelchair.

Your husband/partner might be asked to wait in your presurgery room or in a chair outside the OR until all presurgical preparations are complete. That's because the OR is a sterile environment and a small area with lots of people (nurses, surgical technicians, surgeon, assistant surgeon, pediatrician, anesthetist, nursery nurse, etc.) who need to be sure there's no risk for contamination of the surgical area. It's also important that your spinal or epidural anesthesia is working well before guests are allowed in the room. In the rare event that you need general anesthesia, your husband or partner will not be allowed to sit with you in the OR. Don't worry; your nurse won't forget your partner, and as long as everything is proceeding normally, she'll make sure he or she is by your side before surgery starts.

What Happens in the Operating Room

The operating room (OR) will be cold and bright, but your nurse will cover you with warm blankets. You'll sit on the edge of a narrow OR bed (sometimes called the operating table), while your anesthetist prepares for your spinal or epidural anesthesia, asks questions, puts heart, respiratory, and blood pressure monitors on (heart/respiratory monitors will be stickers that attach to your chest and ribs. Monitor leads will snap onto the stickers and feed information to monitoring machines). When she's ready to start, the anesthetist will ask you to bend forward and curl around your tummy. She'll clean your back, numb the skin, and put in your spinal or epidural. After she's injected the medication that will make you numb for surgery, she'll help you lie down quickly. Spinal anesthesia starts to work within a very short period of time. Don't worry that you can't move your legs. Your nurse and doctor will do the moving for you.

Spinal anesthesia starts to work within a very short period of time. Don't worry that you can't move your legs. Your nurse and doctor will do the moving for you.

Then your nurse will put a Foley catheter into your bladder to keep it empty and out of the way during surgery. It also helps staff monitor your urinary output to make sure your body is processing fluids properly. The catheter stays in for twelve to twenty-four hours after surgery so you don't have to get up to go to the bathroom right away and so your doctor and nurse will know that your bladder is working well after surgery.

Your legs will be secured to the bed with a thick Velcro strap so they won't flop off the bed during surgery. Your arms will rest on arm boards and may or may not be covered lightly with Velcro straps. These straps aren't meant to strap you down, but to keep you from falling or involuntarily touching the sterile surgical area. In some hospitals, mom is able

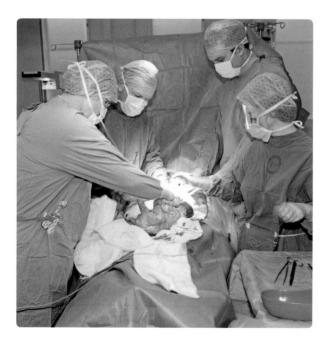

A team of health care providers will work together during your C-section. It will include your OB/GYN, an anesthetist, usually a second surgeon to assist your doctor, plus a surgical nurse, circulating nurse, nursery nurse, and possibly a pediatrician.

to hold her baby in the OR while surgery is still going on. In that case, arm straps aren't used at all.

You may have compression boots placed on your lower legs, which are attached to a machine that repeatedly inflates and deflates the boots. This is done to make sure that the blood in your lower legs is properly circulating to lower your risk of developing blood clots in your legs. These boots will stay on until you're able to get up and walk on your own. Some women love the boots' massagelike feeling, but some women find them hot and confining. Tell your nurse if you're uncomfortable and she can adjust them.

An electrocautery grounding pad will be applied to your thigh. This is a big adhesive pad attached to a lead that connects to an electrocautery unit. The grounding pad prevents electrical burns during surgery. Cautery is a surgical tool and technique used to seal blood vessels to keep bleeding to a minimum. If you notice a burning smell during surgery, that's the cautery.

The blanket covering your abdomen will be turned down, and your nurse will scrub your abdomen, ribs, and thighs with a surgical cleaning solution. You probably won't feel this, but if you do, don't worry that it means you'll feel pain during surgery. Your anesthesia will block pain but may not block sensations of pressure and movement. Once your scrub is finished, your doctor will cover your abdomen with a blue paper and plastic surgical drape. The end closest to your face will be clipped to block your view of surgery. Although you might be curious about what's going on, most women don't want to watch their surgery. Your surgeon might drop the

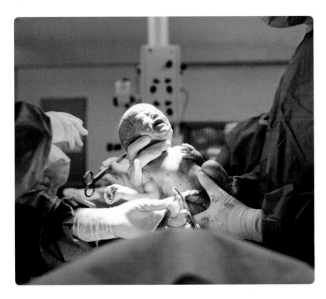

Your baby's birth time is marked at the precise moment when his body is completely out of yours.

hand instruments to your doctor, and a team of nurses will be ready to receive your baby and assist with whatever is needed during surgery.

The surgeon and anesthesiologist will check to make sure that your anesthesia is working properly before making the incision. They may ask you questions such as, "Can you feel this? Does it feel like a pinch?"

Your anesthetist's job is to make sure you're not in pain during surgery and evaluate your vital signs. Very rarely the spinal or epidural anesthesia he administers won't be adequate to cover surgical pain. It might be one-sided, not strong enough, or simply not working well enough. When that happens, he'll attempt to administer a better-functioning spinal, use IV sedation, or general anesthesia (you'll go to sleep). General anesthesia is not the preferred anesthesia for C-sections because the drugs can cross the placenta and anesthetize baby.

drape when the baby is coming out so you can see him or her right away.

Once your drape is in place and the surgical team is assembled, your spouse or partner will be escorted into the OR to a chair next to your head where he can touch your hand or face. He may be able to stand up and watch your surgery (that's up to your anesthetist) and photograph your baby, though it isn't always a good idea. Surgery can be shocking if you're not used to it, and it makes some people woozy.

What Happens during Surgery

During surgery, your anesthetist will sit by your head to monitor your vital signs and administer pain-relieving and antibiotic medications. Your doctor and an assistant surgeon will stand on either side of your belly. A scrub nurse or technician will

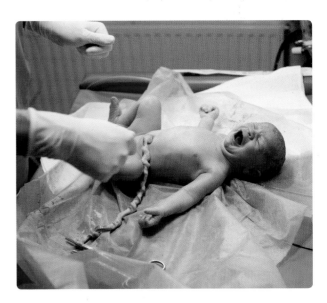

Your baby will be transferred to a radiant warmer, dried off, and assessed for how well she's transitioning to life outside the uterus.

It is associated with greater complications, plus mom misses the birth. It's only used when there's no time for a spinal or the spinal just doesn't work.

Surgery starts when an incision about 3 to 4 inches (7.5 to 10 cm) long is made horizontally just above your pubic hairline. On rare occasions an incision is made vertically. Once she's cut through the skin, your surgeon will use a variety of instruments to methodically work through the layers of adipose (fat) and abdominal muscles and into the peritoneal cavity that contains your uterus, bladder, and intestines. An incision will be made through the uterus and amniotic membrane.

At this point, you'll hear loud suctioning noises as amniotic fluid and blood is vacuumed from the uterus and abdominal cavity. Then you'll feel a lot of tugging and pressure as your doctor reaches inside the uterus and maneuvers your baby out through the uterine incision. This is an intense feeling that some women find uncomfortable but not painful. These weird sensations will be brief, and the next thing you know, your baby is born.

From the start of your C-section to birth will usually take about ten to fifteen minutes. Once the baby is out, your doctor will deliver the placenta and begin the process of closing your uterus. The rest of your surgery will take approximately twenty minutes or longer as each layer of tissue is carefully stitched closed. The skin layer will be closed with sutures (stitches), glue, tape, staples, or a combination of these.

From the start of your C-section to birth will usually take about ten to fifteen minutes.

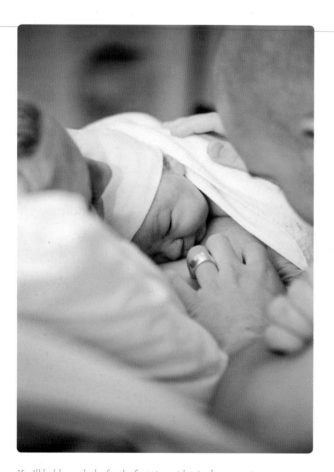

You'll hold your baby for the first time either in the operating room or in the postpartum/recovery room. You should be able to breastfeed too, though movement right after surgery will be challenging for a few hours. Your partner and nurse will help you hold and position your baby comfortably until you're able to do it by yourself.

THE REAL DEAL: *Take Your Time*

Even though a happy event is to be celebrated, a C-section is still major abdominal surgery. Parents are caught off guard by how much recovery time is needed. They plan for a birthday party experience but then discover they're in pain, exhausted, and having a hard time coping and healing. C-sections are not the same as a vaginal birth, and you shouldn't push yourself to recover as quickly as you would from a vaginal birth.

Many women feel pretty good within a day or so of surgery. But some women experience nausea, pain, and fatigue, which makes it very difficult to be hands-on with a newborn. Don't try to be a superhero. Take your pain meds and medications for nausea if necessary. Walk whenever you can and breastfeed your baby if possible. After that . . . rest, rest, rest. That's the best recipe for healing. Your body needs to recover. If you resist, your body will retaliate with slower healing.

This is where dad or your partner comes in. Let him or her take charge of baby. Leave everything other than mandatory personal care and breastfeeding up to your spouse, partner, nurse, family, and/or doula until you're feeling better. Most women feel good within days of surgery.

Think carefully about how many people visit you in the hospital and during your first few days at home. Even though it's a birthday, it's really not an ideal time to be having a party. No matter how well you're healing, you'll be in pain and your body will be working hard to knit your tissues back together, and on making milk.

Don't overtax your resources by over-entertaining. Your focus should be on bonding, healing, and breastfeeding. Invite a few essential family members to visit briefly in the hospital, but wait a week or so to introduce your baby to the rest of your family and friends. Take time to heal properly so you don't have complications later on.

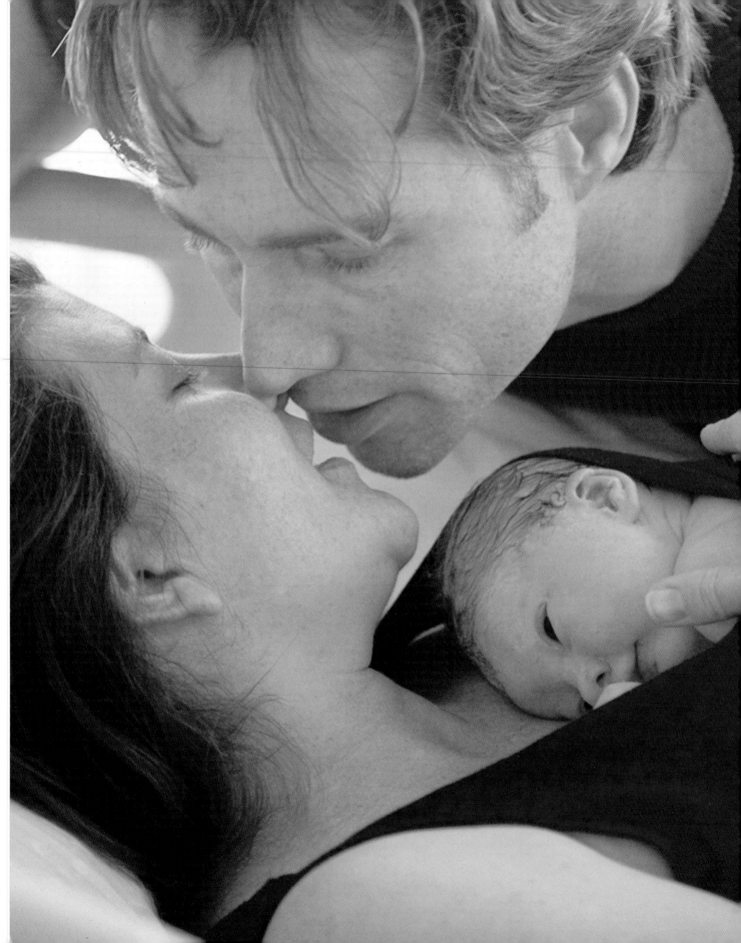

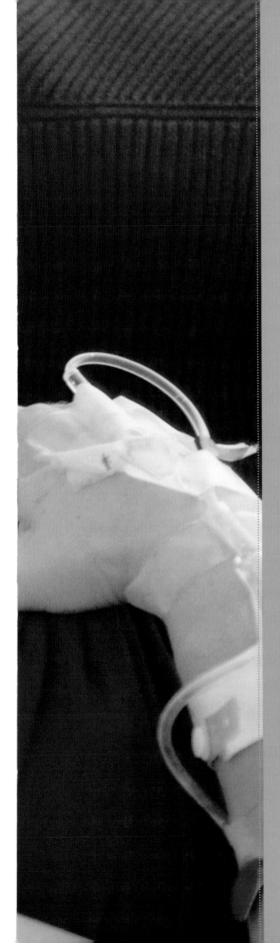

CHAPTER 9

Unplanned Cesarean Birth in a Hospital

What it is, why it may or may not be right for you, pros and cons, and how to prepare for this labor path

Most primary, or first-time, Cesarean sections come as a surprise. Parents head into their final days of pregnancy and toward labor and delivery with all eyes on a vaginal birth. They've written their birth plan, taken their childbirth education classes, practiced their breathing and relaxation techniques, studied up on epidurals, and organized the perfect labor support team. But then something unforeseen happens. The list of unexpected occurrences that might mean birth takes place in the operating room instead of a delivery room is long. Sometimes the reason is an honest-to-goodness, no-doubt-about-it emergency. More often, however, it's not quite as black and white and, sometimes, parents are left wondering why mom needed a C-section at all.

We've broken down the common reasons why women have unplanned C-sections into three categories: nonurgent, urgent, and emergency.

Inside Information

Frequently women have C-sections and don't really understand why they needed one—and some-times they have C-sections they didn't need at all. Considering how high our C-section rate is, and new information indicating health risks associated with them, it's important that women understand when and why they need a C-section and when and why they really don't.

When a baby or mother is in big trouble, C-sections are lifesaving events, and thank goodness we have them. Sometimes, however, C-sections are done when more time or other techniques might be safe, successful, and a better option. How do you know the difference? By asking questions at the time the C-section is recommended. Hopefully you've established a trusting relationship with your health care provider during your pregnancy that allows for open communication and mutual under-standing. If your doctor says, "We need to do this C-section now and there's no time to wait," you want to be sure you can trust him or her. If the circumstances indicate baby or mom's life is in dan-ger, then a C-section is probably your best option. If your provider says, however, "I think it's a good idea," you want to be sure you can talk through other ideas, too.

Fairly often patients hear doctors say, "I can't guarantee you'll deliver vaginally and we don't want to put you through a long labor, so we might as well do a C-section now." Is baby in trouble? Is mom in danger? If the answer is "no," then why do you need a guarantee so badly that having major surgery is a better option? What factors are present that prevent you from proceeding toward a vagi-nal delivery, guaranteed or not? If you can't get satisfactory answers to these questions, then maybe having a C-section isn't really necessary.

Sometimes doctors recommend C-sections in situations that midwives do not, for example, a labor that's taking longer than expected. But if there are no other problems going on, other than a slowpoke pace, then what's the rush? Sometimes a midwife or doctor hasn't been trained to manage a particular birth situation, even though a vaginal birth is possible (for example, with the use of differ-ent manual techniques, an operative vaginal delivery with forceps or vacuum, or other procedures). Maybe his or her partner, however, is trained in that particular technique that would keep you out of the OR. Maybe your doctor is nervous about an on-the-fence situation and feels more comfortable with a C-section delivery. Maybe a consultation with another provider or agreeing to try other spe-cific techniques might help your doctor feel more comfortable.

What if your doctor says she wants to do a C-section, but you're not convinced you want or need one? Ask questions. State your concerns. Ask for more information.

If it's a serious emergency, don't mess around. If it's not, however, start negotiating. Tell your doctor you want to try other options or give labor more time instead. Set specific goals, for example, "Let's wait two more hours and see if anything changes."

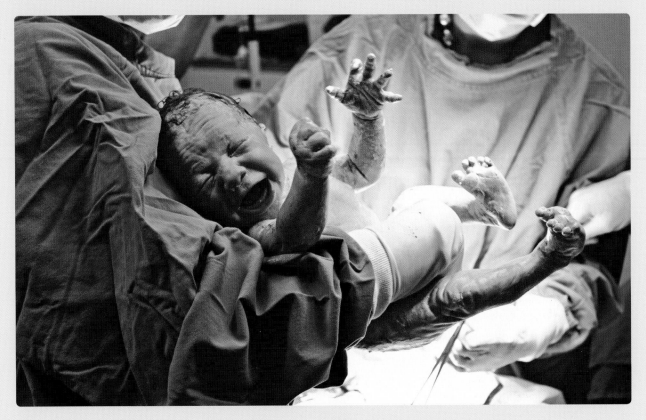

When there's a real emergency, doctors can get babies delivered by C-section and into the arms of health care providers trained to care for sick babies in less than ten to fifteen minutes.

If it's a situation where your doctor says, "I can't guarantee a vaginal birth," tell him or her you don't need a guarantee to keep trying for one. If your doctor says, "I don't think you're going to dilate any further or your baby is too big to descend further," ask whether there's any reason why you can't keep trying. If your baby is not showing any signs of distress and mom isn't showing signs of infection, or other problems, then why not keep going?

If your doctor insists and you still don't agree, ask to speak with the doctor and nurse manager who are the heads of the department. This is a rare and unusual situation, but when it happens, it's an indication that communication and trust between provider and patient has broken down and needs to be remedied before mom or baby's health is compromised.

The most important thing about your birth is not the method of delivery but the health of mother and baby. Keep that in mind when you're negotiating and remember, your doctor or midwife is there to provide the benefit of his or her expertise, but the decisions you make and the risks you take are ultimately your own.

What Is Dad's/Your Partner's Role in an Unplanned C-Section?

If your unplanned C-section is done for nonemergency reasons that don't require general anesthesia, your partner can most likely accompany you to the OR, sit by your side, and provide emotional support. If baby is healthy upon delivery, he or she can be wrapped and placed in your partner's arms, just like with a planned C-section. If baby is not healthy, however, and needs intensive care, your partner's role is to provide mom with emotional support.

If baby has to leave the OR and go to the nursery for more medical treatment, your partner might have the option to accompany baby to the nursery or stay in the OR with mom. Once he leaves the OR, however, he might not be allowed to come back in because that could potentially compromise the OR's sterile atmosphere, and staff members might not be available to accompany him. Different hospitals have different policies about that, and parents should ask about them in advance. If dad decides to stay with mom, he can go to the nursery once she's stable and recovering.

Nurses and/or the pediatrician will come to see the parents and give them all the information that's available about baby's health status. Depending on mom's status, her partner's job may be to act as a liaison between the nursery, mom, and the rest of the family until it's appropriate for them to see the baby. If baby's care is stable, dad should also spend as much time as possible near baby to begin the bonding process. Having a family member present in the nursery is important so the nurses there can begin the teaching process that goes along with caring for any newborn, especially ones who are medically challenged.

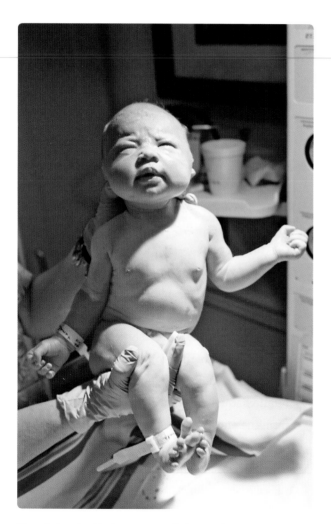

If your baby is healthy, he can go into dad's arms during the remainder of your C-section. If not, he'll receive medical care in the operating room and may be transferred to the NICU.

Care of Baby and Mom Immediately after Delivery

Postpartum procedures for mom are the same no matter what type of C-section you have (planned or unplanned), though recovery may feel a bit different. See chapter 8 for a complete description of what to expect during the immediate postpartum period. Here's how postpartum care differs for mom and baby following an unplanned C-section:

Baby care after an unplanned C-section depends on baby's condition.

- If healthy, baby can go into dad's arms during surgery, and if mom is also healthy, can go back to her recovery and postpartum room. Baby care will then be the same as if mom had a planned C-section or vaginal delivery.
- If baby has complications, he or she will be resuscitated initially in the OR and may go to the NICU while mom is still having surgery. If there's a choice, dad has the option of going to the NICU or staying with mom. It's a good idea if mom and dad/partner discuss this scenario during pregnancy. Some parents feel the best place for dad is near his baby's side, but some feel his role is to support mom, especially if baby or mom's health is compromised. There is no single answer for what to do here. Dad/partner may want to ask mom and baby's health care provider teams for direction about where he is most needed.

Mom's recovery may be a little tougher if she had a C-section after labor; after pushing; if she had a vertical instead of horizontal scar (rare); or if she received general anesthesia.

- If her C-section followed labor, mom might be more exhausted from the hours of contractions she experienced prior to surgery.
- If it followed pushing, she may have a sore bottom as well as a sore abdomen.
- If she has a vertical or very large incision or had any other surgical procedure done at the time of her C-section (for example, a hysterectomy), she may require more recovery and healing time and more pain medication.
- If she had general anesthesia, she may be in more pain than if she had a spinal or epidural injected with long-acting pain medication. She may feel groggy and nauseated from the effects of anesthesia and may need more pain medication and antinausea medication than if she had a spinal or epidural.

The remainder of her recovery and postpartum period will be the same as with a planned C-section (see chapter 8).

HOW TO PREPARE FOR AN UNPLANNED C-SECTION

Prepare for an unplanned C-section? Sounds kind of counterintuitive, right? But the fact of the matter is that as long as one in three women in the United States is statistically giving birth via C-section, even if you don't plan on having one yourself, it may be a good idea to prepare for one—just in case. It's better to be informed about C-sections rather than be completely surprised and blindsided if you unexpectedly find yourself having one. Better to understand the risks, benefits, and procedure now rather than when you're grappling with contractions or an emergency situation. Here's how:

- Read up on C-sections, even if you don't anticipate having one, and even if you have your heart set on a natural delivery.

- Take a childbirth class that discusses C-sections in depth.

- Talk to your health care provider about any potential situations that could arise where you would need an unplanned Cesarean delivery.

- Tour the labor and delivery unit of the hospital where you'd be most likely to have an unplanned Cesarean delivery.

- Make a backup birth plan that helps you think through how to approach a Cesarean delivery if you need to have one at the last minute.

- Think through the plans that you'd need to have in place at home if you were to have an unplanned Cesarean delivery. For instance, if you have older children or pets, do you have someone who could care for them while you're

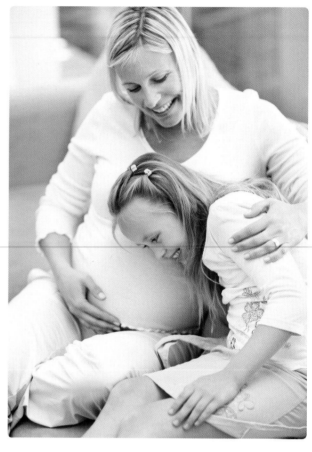

Recovery from a C-section requires three to four days in the hospital. Make sure you have a "just in case" plan for taking care of older children at home, should the situation arise.

in the hospital? (Remember that you'd be in the hospital for approximately four days after a Cesarean, as opposed to the typical two days after a vaginal birth.) Think through the support network you'd need at home for the first few weeks after your delivery, as you'd be recovering from a major abdominal surgery. For instance, you may not be able to lift your baby, get in and out of bed on your own, drive, or do housework for a week to several weeks after your C-section.

The Role of Pain Medications after an Unplanned Cesarean

Many women worry about the pain medications given for postpartum pain management after a Cesarean delivery, especially how they'll affect the baby if mom is breastfeeding. Rest assured that the medications your nurse or health care provider will give you for pain have been approved by the American Academy of Pediatrics as being safe for breastfeeding moms, as long as they're taken as they're prescribed.

Don't feel like you need to be a martyr for your baby's sake—you've just had major abdominal surgery, and now isn't the time to refuse pain medication. Also, consider that you will likely need to take the pain medication to function enough to care for your baby—you want to be comfortable enough to get out of bed, change a diaper, and feed the baby, and you won't be able to do so if you're in pain.

Don't feel like you need to be a martyr for your baby's sake—now isn't the time to refuse pain medication.

There's strong consensus in the medical community that the benefits of breastfeeding far outweigh any risks associated with these pain medications (again, as long as they're taken in the amounts and for the time period prescribed by your health care provider). However, some women feel more comfortable taking steps to minimize their babies' exposure to pain medications while breastfeeding, such as breastfeeding just before they take their pain medication. (The pain medication will be at its highest level in your body in the hour or two after you take it.)

Dealing with Feelings of Disappointment after an Unplanned C-Section

Many, though certainly not all, women find that—once their babies are safely in their arms and they've had a chance to process their labor and delivery experience—they feel deeply disappointed that their babies were delivered via Cesarean section. Some women feel that they somehow "failed," because their bodies were unable to deliver their babies "naturally."

Others feel that they were unduly robbed of the experience of a natural birth. Some feel that they weren't able to immediately bond with their babies, because they were in too much pain to hold their babies or breastfeed immediately, or because they were feeling "off" because of pain medication. These are all valid, normal feelings, especially if your birth didn't go the way you'd hoped or planned. It's important to acknowledge these feelings and to talk about them with your partner, your health care provider, and other women who've had

THE REAL DEAL: *Have No Fear*

Cesarean sections are almost always a lot quicker and easier than patients anticipate. Many parents come to the hospital determined to never have a C-section, filled with anxiety that a C-section is their worst-case scenario. They go through a long labor or pushing process and then go to the OR expecting a nightmare situation. Instead, the vast majority of women find their C-section experience to be quick (they're back in their rooms with a baby in their arms in less than an hour), relatively painless (during surgery at least), and wonder why they were so afraid. As C-section is the most commonly performed surgery done in the United States; doctors are very, very skilled at it; and it is usually a very smooth operation.

Avoiding a C-section is usually the best plan, but when it has to happen, you can rest assured that it probably won't be horrible, you won't suffer, it won't ruin your birth experience, and your baby will be fine. Yes, you can still hold and breastfeed your baby. Yes, you'll be in more pain, but you'll receive pain medication that will make you comfortable. Yes, your recovery will take a little longer, but you'll be up and around within a day or so after surgery and within a week or two, you'll be able to take care of your baby with minimal help.

A C-section isn't ideal, but it's also not the end of the world (though losing your life, health, or baby would be). It doesn't mean you failed, that you're less of a woman or a wimp. It means you needed an alternative to have the best birth possible.

While we work toward reducing the C-section rate, let's also work toward making C-sections less frightening and anxiety- and guilt-provoking than they are for some women. Bottom line: If you need one, you'll probably be glad you had one, and you're almost certainly going to be fine.

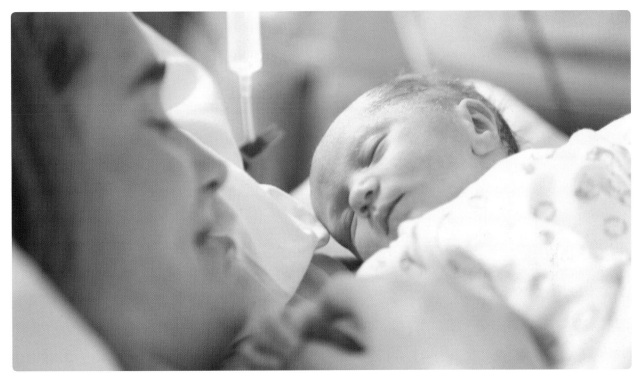

C-sections are the most commonly performed surgery in the United States and for most women, they're quick and easy procedures. Barring any complications, you'll have a baby in your arms in under an hour.

an unplanned C-section. Allow yourself a "grieving period" to get through your emotions, especially if your birth simply didn't go the way you dreamed it would. Keep in mind that birth can be unpredictable and that—in the end—everyone's goal is a healthy mom and baby, by the safest means possible. Assuming that you chose a health care provider whose expertise you inherently trust, you can rest assured that you and your health care provider did what was best for you and your baby, based on the information you had available at the time.

If you find that you can't get past your feelings of disappointment, ask to have a "birth review" with your health care practitioner, so you can better understand the reasons behind your unplanned Cesarean. And if you worry that you have strong feelings of anger or depression that could potentially be signs of postpartum depression, talk to your health care provider and your partner about getting the care and support you need, because you and your baby both deserve to have a happy, healthy start to your new life together.

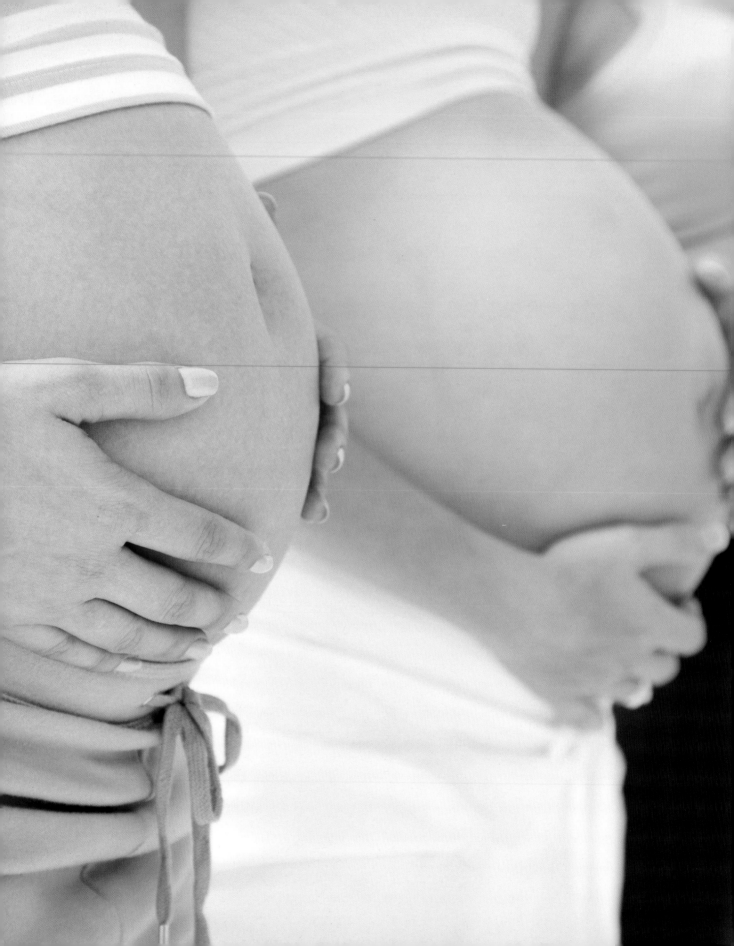

CHAPTER 10

Managing the Pain of Labor

Your labor tool kit,
from rice socks to spinal blocks

Whether you're leaning toward a drug-free delivery or you'd like to get an epidural at the first possible moment, there are plenty of ways to make your labor more comfortable.

Right now, you're doing the most important thing you can do when it comes to managing labor pain—you're educating yourself about what to expect. Going into labor with a good understanding of what's happening helps take the fear away from the process. If you're afraid, you're more likely to tense up, causing your body more pain. But equipped with knowledge about the labor process, you'll be more likely to relax and work with your body rather than resisting the process. For that reason, we'll begin this chapter with an overview of the stages of labor, so you know what to expect and when. You'll also find a range of tried-and-true tips for handling the pain of labor, from breathing to massage, meditation, movement, and more.

THE STAGES OF LABOR

Knowing what's happening to your body at each stage of the game makes a big difference. Here's a quick overview of the stages of labor and what you may be feeling along the way:

The First Stage: Early Labor and Active Labor

Early Labor

"Early" labor can also be defined as "prodromal" labor, which in medical terms means "not yet in active labor." Don't be alarmed by women who swear that their labors were several days long. Sure, women may feel regular contractions for several days, but labor itself doesn't really kick off until regular, painful contractions are dilating the cervix. For the most part, labor starts and progresses, and finishes with a lovely birth. But sometimes it just can't seem to get going, which results in a long prodromal stage, with lots of contractions that hurt but aren't all that close together and aren't helping your cervix to dilate. No one knows why this happens, but if it happens to you, you need to be in touch with your health care provider to try to stop the contractions or speed them up. (If you find that you're unable to sleep, sometimes induced sleep with a narcotic can be helpful. You either wake up in good labor or find that the contractions subside for a while and come back later.)

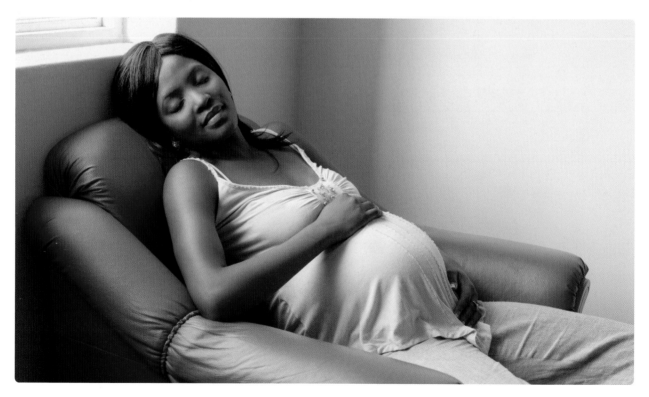

Visualization techniques should be practiced regularly during pregnancy so you'll be ready to use this tool during your labor. Choose an image that makes you feel safe, calm, and peaceful—a.k.a. your "happy place."

In early labor, you may feel contractions that last anywhere from thirty to sixty seconds, coming anywhere from five to twenty minutes apart. When labor first begins, your contractions may feel more like consistently strong menstrual cramps. Gradually they'll increase in intensity, coming closer and closer together. These contractions are beginning to dilate your cervix. Your water may break at the onset of labor, or it may stay intact until the very end stages of labor. You may notice your mucus plug or even some bloody show in early labor.

What to Do: Take advantage of early labor to rest, relax, and prepare for what's ahead. If you can, lie down on your side for a while and take a nap. Or take a warm bath, read a book or magazine, watch a television show, or listen to music to take your mind off labor. If you can't rest, try going for a walk or going about your daily activities. Try to ignore your contractions for as long as you can. With your health care provider's okay, this is also a good time to have a healthy snack or meal—it may be your last chance to eat until after the baby's born.

Active Labor

During active labor your contractions become much stronger, longer, and closer together. You'll have little time to rest in between contractions, and you may be feeling a lot more pain and pressure. By the end of active labor, your cervix will dilate up to ten centimeters, and you'll be ready to start pushing!

What to Do: Active labor is a great time to try some of the tips and tricks in this chapter.

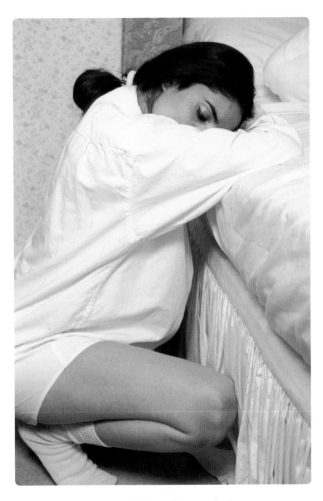

Changing positions frequently during labor can facilitate an easier labor and help baby ease down into the birth canal. Try squatting, leaning on the bed, walking, turning side to side, or use a birthing ball.

The Second Stage: Pushing and the Birth of Your Baby!

Once your cervix has dilated to ten centimeters, you're ready to start pushing! It won't be long now before you'll be holding your baby in your arms. This stage of labor can last anywhere from twenty minutes up to three hours or more. First-time moms generally have a longer pushing phase, while mothers who've previously given birth often

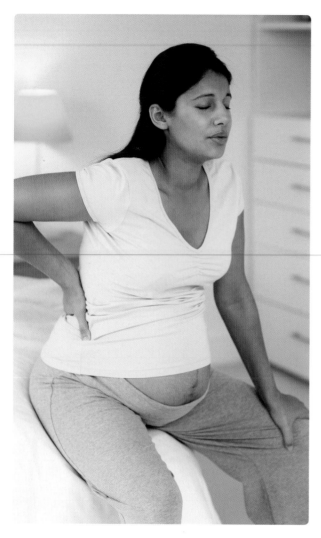

Slow, deep breathing is among the most effective pain management techniques you can use. It's not so important to use a specific breathing technique or pattern—just focus on your breath and relax.

have a much shorter second stage of labor. If your pushing phase lasts longer than two to three hours, it is considered to be a prolonged second stage, which is fine if your health care provider feels comfortable with it. Most health care providers will reevaluate after two hours, but for a first-time mom having a baby with an epidural, three hours

of pushing is considered normal. You may feel pressure on your rectum and a strong urge to push. This stage ends with the birth of your baby.

What to Do: Who says you need to stay in one position to push your baby? Do what works for you. Try using squat bars or birthing stools, or getting on all fours. A more upright position will allow you to use gravity to your advantage to help push the baby out. For more on labor positions, see the "Movement" section in this chapter.

The Third Stage: Delivery of the Placenta

While you're most likely holding your newborn and bonding, your health care provider will help deliver the placenta. Many women hardly even notice this stage of delivery because they're so focused on their babies! It takes about five to thirty minutes to deliver the placenta, during which you may feel contractions and even chills or shakiness. Your health care provider may ask you to push at a certain point. If you'd like, you can ask to see your placenta after it's delivered—it can be a truly unique experience to see the organ that's helped nourish your baby all this time.

NONMEDICAL WAYS TO EASE PAIN

There are plenty of drug-free ways to manage your pain. Here are some that we like best:

Breathing. You don't necessarily have to subscribe to a particular style of breathing, such as the "hee-hee-hoo-hoo" breathing technique made popular by Lamaze. It's less important to breath in a particular way and more important to simply focus on your natural breathing. Tuning in to your breathing acts as a meditation of sorts, because it calms and focuses your mind, relaxing your whole body in the process. Plus, the increased oxygen flow will help give you an extra boost of energy.

Birthing balls. The great thing about birthing balls is that you can use them to strengthen your legs and core before and after labor, as well as during the delivery. Sitting on a birthing ball can help take some of the pressure off your back while encouraging you to relax and open up your pelvic region.

Contraction exercise. Sit on a birthing ball positioned at the foot of a bed and lean your head and chest into the bed, with your arms outstretched across the bed. (You can also try leaning over the ball while you're kneeling on the bed.) Ask your doula, partner, or labor coach to press the palms of his or her hands firmly against your hips, pressing them down into the birthing ball. Be sure to let your coach know when a contraction is beginning and ending, so he or she can apply the right amount of pressure throughout—you'll be amazed at how much relief you'll feel!

Birthing stools. A birthing stool, which is essentially a U-shaped stool for a laboring woman to sit on, can be one of your best tools during the later stages of labor. It allows you to sit on the stool in a squatting position, using gravity to ease the baby down the birth canal while taking the pressure off your legs.

Cool or warm compresses. Cool or warm compresses can do wonders for your muscles—and your mood. They can be as simple as a washcloth dipped in a bowl of ice water (for your face), or run under a warm faucet (for your back or your perineum when baby's crowning). Or try a "rice sock," which can quickly be warmed up in a microwave. A frozen water bottle or a frozen pack of peas works great as a cold compress. Also try a hot water bottle or a heating pad—this feels great against the lower back if you're having a lot of back discomfort.

Hypnosis. Hypnosis can help you direct your mind away from the pain of labor and into a state of deep relaxation. If you'd like to learn about hypnosis in labor, you may want to consider taking a class, buying a book on hypnosis, or listening to some CDs. It's a technique that should be practiced regularly and often—well before you're in labor. Some of the more well-known hypnosis programs include the Peaceful Pregnancy Program, HypnoBirthing (as originally coined by Michelle Leclaire O'Neill), the Mongan Method (also known as HypnoBirthing), Hypnobabies, Confident Childbirth (cognitive hypnotherapy), Natal Hypnotherapy, FreshStart, and the GentleBirth program. Many women who've used hypnosis in labor report that they felt less pain in labor, had shorter labors, and felt more in control of their birth experiences.

Rice sock. Although you can buy a nice rice sock commercially, it's just as easy to make your own. Simply find a clean tube sock and fill it with uncooked rice. Tie off the end and put it in the microwave for two to three minutes. It'll hold the heat—and relax your muscles—for up to a half an hour. Press it against your lower back or wear it around your neck like a scarf to ease neck and shoulder pain. Alternatively, you can use the rice

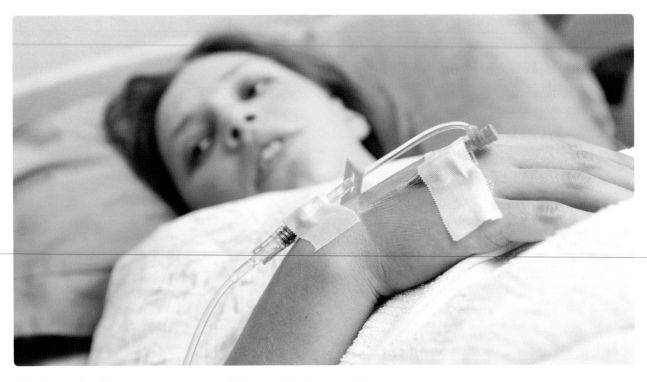

All medication-based pain management options, including an epidural, require an IV.

Opiates and Other Pain Medications

Opiates are often used in labor to "take the edge off" pain for women who've already tried some of the more natural methods such as water, breathing, and massage but aren't quite ready for an epidural. An opiate will not numb the pain like an epidural but can help reduce anxiety and improve a woman's ability to cope with the pain.

Some women just need a touch of pain medication, and the narcotics Stadol and Nubain—opiod agonists/antagonists—are often used. These medications make mom sleepy. Babies get a larger dose of medication when these are used, as generally they are given intravenously and intramuscularly. Rarely, a baby can be lethargic at birth as a result of these medications, in which case the baby will need medication to counteract the effects.

Narcotics should not be used if your health care provider thinks you are going to have your baby within the hour. This would not give your body the time to clear the medication, and your baby would be born with more of it in his or her system. Also, narcotics are not given if there's any question about fetal well-being, as the narcotics can affect the fetal heart rate.

Note: Stadol and Nubain cannot be used in someone who takes methadone because they counteract the results of methadone and can cause instant withdrawal symptoms and seizures in the mother and baby, and even death.

Demerol and morphine are other narcotics that may be used in labor, and although they are a different class of medication, they work similarly to Stadol and Nubain.

Some doctors still do local regional blocks such as pudendal blocks for perineal repair or a forceps delivery, but nowadays the epidural is so common that pudendal blocks are used very infrequently.

Potential side effects of opiates for the mother:

- Nausea

- Vomiting

- Itching

- Dizziness

- Sedation

- Decreased gastric motility

- Loss of protective airway reflexes

- Hypoxia because of respiratory depression

Potential side effects of opiates for the baby:

- Central nervous system depression

- Respiratory depression

- Impaired early breastfeeding

- Altered neurological behavior

- Decreased ability to regulate body temperature

Inside Information

How well do narcotic pain medications work to relieve labor pain? For some women, one dose is all they need to get over a pain roadblock. They relax, their labor progresses, and they don't need anything else.

For most women, however, one dose is not enough. Depending on which medication they receive (it could be fentanyl, Stadol, Nubain, morphine, or Demerol), the first dose might work well for an hour or more. If you need a second dose, it will probably help reduce your pain, but don't expect it to work as well as the first dose did. That's because you'll be further along in labor, your contractions will be stronger, and the narcotic receptors in your body will be filling up. Combine all those factors and the result is that dose number two just isn't as effective as the first dose.

If you need a third dose, "fuggedaboudit"—you probably need an epidural instead. If your nurse, midwife, or doctor thinks your baby will be born within an hour or two, then using narcotics isn't appropriate. These drugs cross the placenta and baby gets a dose, too, which could cause respiratory depression if he's born before it clears his system. That's why your providers might tell you, "It's too late for a shot, but there's still time for an epidural."

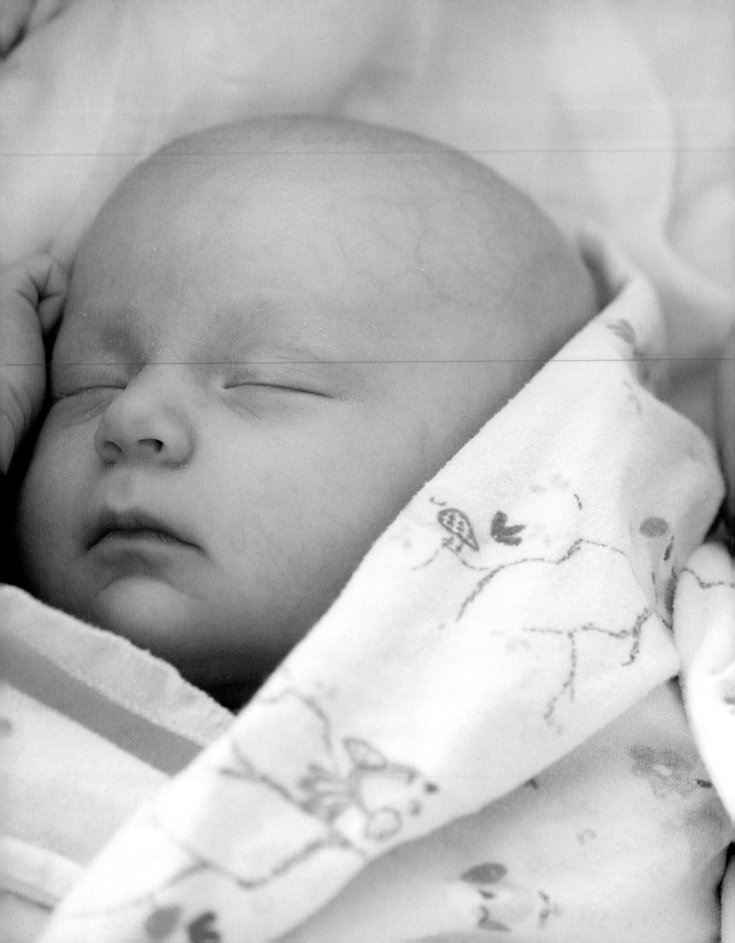

CHAPTER 11

Creating Your Birth Plan

Nailing down your wish list, and what to do when things don't go according to plan

Why write a birth plan? It's a great way to get your thoughts and feelings about your baby's birth down on paper. It's a helpful tool for thinking through the various scenarios that may present themselves during your baby's birth, so that you can educate yourself about the pros and cons of each situation before you're simultaneously dealing with labor and delivery. And it's a great communication tool to help ensure that your partner/labor coach, health care provider, and you are all on the same page (and if not, what you can do about it and/or how you need to realign your plans).

But here's what it's *not*: Your birth plan is *not* a contract between you and your labor team. It's not a promise for how your labor and delivery will unfold. Many health care providers advise that you think of it more as a wish list of how you would prefer things to unfold, if possible. But you need to keep in mind that labor and delivery can be unpredictable. You and your health care provider may need to shift gears at the last minute for the sake of a healthy mom and baby, and it's a good idea to approach your birth plan with that in mind.

Here's what else it's not: Your birth plan doesn't need to be a novel. Believe it or not, no health care provider has the time or energy to read through a ten-page birth plan. Keep it simple. Keep it clear. Keep it to one or two pages—max. And keep in mind that babies don't read birth plans: Sometimes the plan will simply have to change.

CREATING YOUR BIRTH PLAN

Before you sit down to write your birth plan, spend time thinking very broadly about your baby's birth. Think through the big picture before you start getting into any specifics. You may even want to pull out a journal or a notebook and write free-form about what you envision for your baby's birth.

After you've done this, you can begin nailing down specifics. Here are some questions and considerations to think through:

- Who will be present? (Your partner? Your mother or mother-in-law? Siblings? Your friend? A doula? A midwife? An obstetrician?)

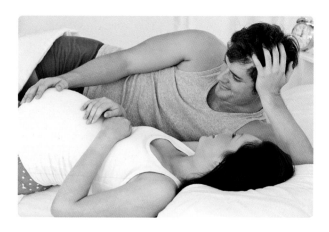

Creating a birth plan with your partner is a great way to start parenting together. It gives you a chance to talk about your goals and hopes for your child and techniques you'll use to achieve them.

- Where do you want to be during the early stages of your labor? (Taking a walk? Relaxing at home? At the hospital? At a birth center?)

- What type of environment would you like for your baby's delivery? (Low lights? Music playing? Privacy? Quiet calm, or a more energetic coaching style?)

- What's your birthing style? Are you anticipating a home birth, a birth center birth, a drug-free hospital delivery, a hospital delivery with an epidural, a VBAC, or a planned Cesarean? Do you have any health conditions that would require a hospital delivery?

- How do you plan to cope with the pain of labor? (Breathing? Hypnosis? Meditation? Pain medications? A tub full of warm water?)

- What tools do you hope to have available to help you get through labor? (A birthing ball? Squat bars? A birthing stool? A birthing tub? Hot and warm compresses? A masseuse? Narcotics? An epidural?)

- How strongly do you feel about being able to eat or drink during labor?

- How strongly do you feel about being able to move around freely during labor?

- How do you feel about fetal monitoring? (Would it reassure you that your baby is doing fine or would it make you overly anxious and restrict you to your bed?)

- How do you feel about having an IV?

- How do you feel about frequent vaginal exams? (Do you want frequent updates on how your cervix is dilating, or do you believe that you'll know best when it's time to push?)

- What if your health care provider wants to do an episiotomy, or use forceps or vacuum extraction, to help get the baby out?

- If you are having a home or birth center birth, what emergency plans are in place for transporting you and your baby to a hospital?

- What are your hopes for after baby's birth, in terms of rooming in, breastfeeding, nursery care, circumcision, and so on?

General Tips on Expressing Your Preferences

The American Pregnancy Association advises against using phrases such as "We don't want" in favor of more positive phrasing such as "We hope to avoid" or "We anticipate," so that your birth plan doesn't come off as a "list of demands" but rather as a clear expression of your preferences.

It's a good idea to do a general gut check to see whether the specific items in your birth plan align with the overall big picture that you envision for your baby's birth. For instance, if you really want to have a natural birth, have you thought about giving birth at a birth center or at home, or having a doula present at your birth?

Go through your ideal scenario first. But don't forget to also think through how you would handle any complications that might arise, which might require you to deviate from your ideal birth plan.

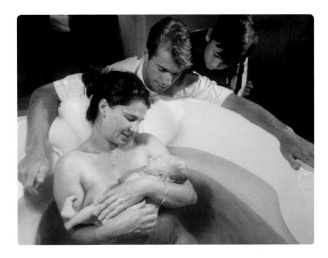

Decide who you want to attend the birth well in advance of labor. Choose only the people who will support you and benefit the most from seeing your baby come into the world.

Who Should Be in the Delivery Room with You?

Is your mother-in-law asking to be present at the baby's birth? What about your best friend, your oldest child, or your sister? You'll definitely want to think through how your extended circle of family and friends fits into your birth plan, and how to help them feel included while still respecting your (and your partner's) own needs for privacy and rest.

When thinking about whom to include at your baby's birth, look into your hospital or birth center's policies on the number of people allowed in the labor and delivery room. Some hospitals make you petition for more than two people in your room. If you show up and ask to admit an extra "support person," you may be denied. Also ask about visiting hours and policies for after the baby's birth.

When you're thinking through whom you'd like to have present during your baby's birth, ask yourself:

- Does this person want to be present, and do my partner and I want him or her to be there?
- What role will this person play during labor?
- Will this person be supportive of my wishes and my birth plan?

- Does this person bring something special to the table (for instance, massage skills, labor coaching skills, or a unique ability to communicate well with my health care provider)?

How to deal with too many or unwanted labor supporters without stepping on toes? Make your wishes clear to everyone up front with statements like "We welcome everyone to wait for news of

THE REAL DEAL: *In Your Dreams*

The labor you dream of in your birth plan is more likely to be your second labor rather than your first one. Most first-time parents can't fully appreciate how long and hard labor is. If you've never been through anything like it, it's hard to wrap your mind around just how strenuous it really is. Even parents who've prepared for birth (and maybe seen one before) can't believe it's going to be that challenging for them. Seriously, how hard can it really be? Straight up: Pretty. Darn. Hard. Harder than anything you've ever done before. This doesn't mean you can't still have that unmedicated birth you wanted, but be prepared for it.

Second labors (and thirds, etc.), on the other hand, tend to be shorter, with less pushing and a much faster, smoother second stage. Your body already knows the ropes. That's the labor most first-timers think they're going to have. That's the one they plan on when they're reading magazines, typing up lists, and deciding how labor is going to go.

It's hard to plan for the complete unknown. Add a big whopping dose of flexibility and clear vision to your first-time birth plan so you're not blindsided. Who knows, you might get lucky and have an easier time than you think. But it might be a lot harder than you planned, too. In fact, plan on it.

the baby's delivery in the family waiting room" or "We'll be sure to call you (or send an email/post a message on Facebook) as soon as possible after the baby's birth." What to do when you have unwanted, uninvited visitors in your labor, delivery, or recovery room? Ask your partner, nurse, or health care provider to run interference. They can kindly suggest that your family and friends retire to

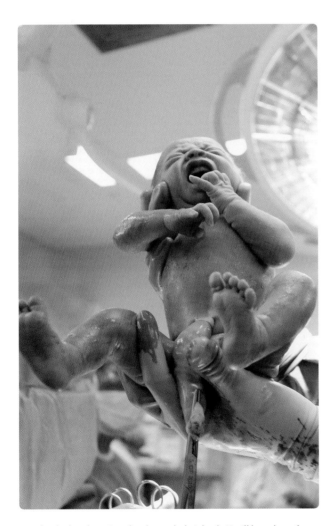

Your birth plan doesn't end with your baby's birth. You'll have lots of decisions to make from what medications and tests your baby will receive, to whether to bank cord blood, to whether to have your son circumcised, and more.

the waiting room or head home, as "mom and baby need to rest." Or hang a sign on your door that says that "Shh . . . mom and baby are sleeping." (Keep in mind that if you end up having a very long labor, you might want to have a few people whom you could call on to relieve your partner or your doula for a while.)

The Birth Plan Doesn't End with the Baby's Birth

Keep in mind that your birth plan doesn't end when your baby is born. There's a lot to think about in the first twenty-four to forty-eight hours after your baby's delivery, on topics such as rooming in, feeding your baby, cord blood banking, circumcision, vaccinations, and more. Here we address a few of the big topics, and we list some of the other decisions you'll be considering after your baby's birth:

Should I bank my baby's cord blood? You've no doubt seen a plethora of ads encouraging you to bank your baby's cord blood. What's the deal? Cord blood is rich in stem cells, which are currently used in transplants for some patients with leukemia, lymphoma, immune deficiencies, and inherited metabolic disorders. Some parents choose to collect a sample of their baby's cord blood and store, or "bank" it, so that it can be used to treat any potential future health care issues for the baby or a close family member. Stem cell technologies are changing rapidly every year, and many believe that although we may not know the potential of using stem cells today, there's much promise for new technologies in the future to treat conditions such as cerebral palsy, stroke, spinal cord injuries, diabetes, and cardiovascular disease.)

Cord blood banking is a personal decision that comes down to your family's medical history and financial situation. From a medical standpoint, cord blood banking is a topic of debate. Many in the health care community believe that donations of stem cells from public banks are as effective as private blood banks. Private blood banking can be expensive, and the odds that your baby, or family

THE REAL DEAL: *Cord Blood Banking*

It doesn't make you a bad mother to just say no to cord blood banking. In fact, we might argue that you *should* say no to private cord blood banking.

The advertising and marketing for private cord blood banking is designed to make parents think if they want the very best for their baby, they have to store her umbilical cord blood in their private bank as insurance against unforeseen diseases she might get down the line. It's a disingenuous tactic, really, because though stem cells in cord blood can be used to treat about 100 genetic diseases, they can almost never be used to treat that baby. That's because if her stem cells contain the gene for the disease she needs treated, then her cord blood can't be used to treat it. Sure, technology may change in the future, but genetics are genetics and no oncologist or pediatrician will recommend using a patient's own blood to treat her genetic disease. Instead she'd need donated stem cells from a public cord blood bank, not the stem cells her family paid thousands of dollars to keep in a private bank.

If parents have the opportunity to collect and donate their baby's umbilical cord blood to a public bank, however, it can create lifesaving miracles for other children with genetic diseases. If the time comes when your child needs help, she can get lifesaving stem cells from the public bank. Bottom line: Private banking = a lot of money for something you probably won't need. Public banking (when and where available) = priceless.

member, will be able to use the cells to treat a future disease are still relatively low.

It's also still not clear how long stored stem cells remain viable. If you choose to bank your baby's cord blood, do your homework on the cord blood banking facilities so you can make an educated choice. You can start with the American Association of Blood Banks at www.aabb.org. Two things to keep in mind as you do your research:

- If you decide to bank your baby's cord blood, choose a company that has used cord blood cells successfully in transplants. Anyone can freeze the blood. The key is being able to thaw it and use it when you need it.

- Shop around for cost. There are plenty of coupons out there, and the companies are competitive—they'll usually offer you a discount or a payment plan option.

Should I get my son circumcised? Circumcision is another very personal decision— and a topic of raging public debate—that you'll want to think through as part of your birth plan. It's a good idea to read as much as you can about the procedure before your baby's birth and discuss it with your partner and your pediatrician before you form your own decision. The American Academy of Pediatricians' (AAP) current policy on circumcision says that "existing scientific evidence demonstrates potential medical benefits of newborn male circumcision; however, these data are not sufficient to recommend routine neonatal circumcision." In other words, the AAP doesn't see enough of a medical reason for

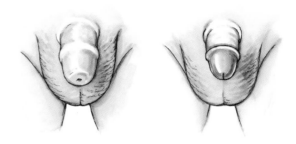

Before and after circumcision: *The foreskin is removed, and the head of the penis is exposed.*

circumcision to recommend that all newborn boys are circumcised. However, it does say that though "the procedure is not essential to the child's current well-being, parents should determine what is in the best interest of the child."

When you make your own decision, read the arguments for and against circumcision and understand what happens during the procedure itself. (We won't go into all of that here, as it's a bit outside the scope of this book. A good source to begin your research is with our own coauthor Jeanne Faulkner's "Ask the Labor Nurse" blog at www.fitpregnancy.com/labor-delivery/ask-labor-nurse/circumcision-back-news.)

THE REAL DEAL: *Circumcision*

Circumcision is medically unnecessary cosmetic surgery. The American Congress of Obstetricians and Gynecologists calls it "elective." The procedure is straightforward and only takes about five minutes. Some babies suffer serious complications, including ones that require a plastic surgeon or a urologist to repair. Many doctors (but not all, despite the AAP's recommendation) use local anesthesia. It wears off and yes, your newborn will be in some pain or discomfort until the area heals, which takes about a week.

Although the AAP doesn't recommend circumcisions, it also hasn't tried to stop them. Religious custom may dictate that boys must be circumcised, or parents want their boys to look like their fathers. But, if you're worried about your son looking different than dad, consider that it might be easier and safer to explain the situation than to make them have surgery.

Although there's some evidence that men in impoverished, developing countries have a lower risk of developing AIDS and other sexually transmitted diseases if they're circumcised, education about unsafe sex and disease and improving hygiene and medical care are far more effective. Circumcision is associated with a lower risk of penile cancer, which happens rarely anyway, in less than 1 out of every 100,000 men. Uncircumcised boys have a higher risk of getting a urinary tract infection in the first year of life, but this overall risk is less than 1 percent.

If you decide to skip the circumcision in the hospital and wait until he's older, know that the procedure is more complicated in an older child because general anesthesia is used, which carries more risk than a local injection.

Bottom line: If you want your son to be circumcised and he has no other health issues, then it will be done, and if you don't, it won't be done. You will be given information about the procedure, and you decide if the benefits outweigh these risks.

When Your Birth Plan Doesn't Go According to Plan

No mother wants to think about anything going wrong during her baby's delivery. But it's important to think through some scenarios now, so that if a complication does arise, you won't be trying to get information and make decisions when you're in pain and when every second counts. If you haven't already read chapter 9 on unplanned Cesarean delivery, we strongly encourage you to do so. It will help you understand and think through what might happen in an emergency situation—even if you think it would never happen to you.

The truth is that no one can say how your labor and delivery will unfold. It's difficult to plan for the unforeseen. So consider your options, but also try to take a look at the other side of the coin. Maybe you plan to have a drug-free birth, but in the throes of labor, you decide that you'd actually like to have an epidural after all. Think through how that scenario might play out and how you feel about it. (That's why, even if you're planning for an unmedicated birth, you may want to read through chapter 5 on having an epidural in a hospital, in case you change your mind. And vice versa—even if you're planning for an epidural, why not read chapters 3 and 4 on unmedicated births, so you know what to expect if you don't end up with an epidural after all.)

No matter how much planning you do, labor is often full of surprises—some pleasant and some, not so much. We've broken down some common if/then scenarios for you to think through as you plan your optimal, but realistic, birth plan.

What if I have preterm labor? There's a big difference between preterm contractions and preterm labor. Lots of women have contractions on and off for weeks (even months) before they go into labor. If those contractions don't change your cervix, then they don't constitute preterm labor. If they do change your cervix and it's before 34 weeks, you might be placed on bed rest and given medications to knock out your contractions. You'll also probably be given a couple shots of a steroid (called betamethasone), which will help your baby's lungs and other organs mature more quickly and increase her chances of survival if she's born prematurely.

If this happens after 34 weeks, your provider probably won't do anything to stop your labor, and you can proceed with your birth plans. Most babies born after 34 weeks do just fine, but some need extra support to maintain their breathing, body temperature, and blood sugar. They might not be mature enough to breastfeed as well as a full-term baby. If your baby needs extra help, she'll probably spend some time in the special care nursery. If she's born at 34 weeks, your baby might not go home with you at two days after birth. A 36- to 37-weeker, on the other hand, probably will.

What if my baby's heart rate drops in labor? A normal baseline heart rate for a baby is between 110 and 160 beats per minute. We expect the heartbeat to vary, accelerating and sometimes decelerating. When baby's heart rate drops, it may or may not signal trouble. Some decelerations are entirely normal. Some signal that baby's umbilical cord might be getting pinched during a contraction or the vagus nerve in his head might be getting stimulated (which causes the heart rate to temporarily slow down). Although this sounds a little scary, it's not usually a cause for worry.

Some types of decelerations are more worrisome than others. For example, if it slows down repetitively *after* several contractions or it slows down and doesn't return to a normal baseline, that's when your nurse, midwife, or doctor might get concerned. There are a lot of easy fixes for decelerations, such as changing mom's position, increasing her hydration, giving her some oxygen, and, if she's getting IV Pitocin, stopping her infusion for a while. Her nurse will check mom's blood pressure, because if it's unusually low, that can affect baby's heart rate. If she's had an epidural and her blood pressure is very low, the nurse might contact the anesthetist to administer medication to increase it while at the same time she gives mom extra IV fluid.

If none of these interventions work, and baby's heart rate continues to look scary, chances are good a C-section will be recommended if vaginal delivery is not imminent. Although we don't always know why babies' hearts act the way they do, we do know that most of the time, they're just fine when they're born.

Troubleshooting Common Conflicts

Sometimes there are road bumps along the way while you are in labor that may or may not affect your outcome but can make things uncomfortable. Here are a few common scenarios we'd like to help you with.

What to do when your husband (or partner, mom, friend, etc.) isn't the best labor partner or when he has a very different birth plan. It happens all the time: Mom wants an epidural—dad wants an all-natural birth. Mom wants a natural birth—her mom (and labor coach) can't stand to see her daughter in pain. Mom planned on having her best friend as her primary labor support, but it turns out she's not actually all that supportive. When that happens, it's time to bring in ancillary support services.

Hash out the plan with your partner well in advance of labor. If you and your partner have really different points of view about what constitutes your perfect birth, you might start negotiating a middle path with a discussion at your provider's office. Maybe dad needs more information or your partner needs to voice her fears. If you really can't come to terms, it might be time to consult a couples counselor. Don't wait until you're in labor to find a solution to this problem and don't let yourself be bullied into someone else's idea of the perfect birth. Sure, you and your partner are in it together, but it's your body that will be going through labor. You'll definitely want to take his or her opinion into consideration, but when the going gets tough, your needs trump his.

If you know that your husband/partner isn't the best choice to provide labor support, don't plan on going it alone. Instead enlist your mother, sister, or best friend or hire a doula. Try not to be resentful that your partner isn't up to the job. Labor support requires a certain amount of tolerance for pain, patience, nerves of steel, and the ability to go the distance hour after hour. Not everyone can do it to the level that many women need. Just find someone else and give your partner another supporting role.

How to get your labor team on board with your plans without making them the "plan police." When you're drawing up your birth plan, you might be tempted to tell your labor team something like this: "Under no circumstances should you let me get an epidural. Even if I beg for one, just say 'no.'" Don't do that. Don't make your labor support team be the "plan police." It's not fair.

Most first-time parents have no idea how labor will affect them. It might be longer, harder, and far more painful than anticipated. Although it's good to make plans about how you want to manage pain or which interventions you do or don't want, your birth plan has to be negotiable, flexible, and work for the benefit of those involved through a rapidly changing scenario.

Try designing a step-by-step process you'll navigate before you change your plans. For example, if you decide you want an epidural, but your plan was to go all natural, you'll first, change positions and wait for ten contractions; second, get in the tub and wait ten contractions; third, consider other forms of pain medication; fourth, get an epidural and be okay with it. Your partner's job is to help you move

through the steps and then help you accept whatever plan you end up with.

Once in a while, a dad, partner, or other labor support person decides to be confrontational, adversarial, and a downright bully when mom decides to do something not included in her birth plan. Dad might try to dominate the situation and intimidate the staff to force mom to stick to the plan. This is a bad situation and usually winds up leaving dad looking like a jerk, mom feeling horrible, and the staff feeling bullied. Don't let this situation play out in your labor room. Talk about how to switch gears before you have to switch them.

How to handle it if you decide you want an epidural after all. The best way to handle any abrupt departure from your birth plan is with acceptance and understanding. Go easy on yourself. About 70 percent of women choose to get epidurals during labor because it's available and they discover that labor is a lot more intense than they'd anticipated. We don't have that many pain options available to us here in the United States, and epidurals are the best way to eliminate the pain most women experience. If you need one and you get one (even if you swore up and down you wouldn't), so be it. Don't beat yourself up about it. It's a medical tool, not a moral judgment, test of character, or a choice between giving birth the right way versus the wrong way.

How do I decide whether I want an episiotomy or a tear? The short answer is this: You don't make that decision, your provider does. Episiotomies are not routinely done anymore. They're saved for extreme situations. Many women won't tear (though most first-timers will), and doing an episiotomy in order to prevent a tear that might or might not happen isn't necessary. When an episiotomy is cut, the perineum sometimes tears further than the episiotomy incision and much further than it would have if left intact.

Episiotomies are not routinely done anymore. They're saved for extreme situations.

Use measures such as hot compresses, oil, and massage to help the perineum stretch gradually. If your provider decides an episiotomy is absolutely necessary, for example, to get baby out more quickly, then so be it. Your provider makes that decision based on the medical situation at hand.

If your perineum does tear, your provider will repair it. It's not any more difficult to stitch up a tear than it is to stitch up an episiotomy. Your bottom will heal well either way.

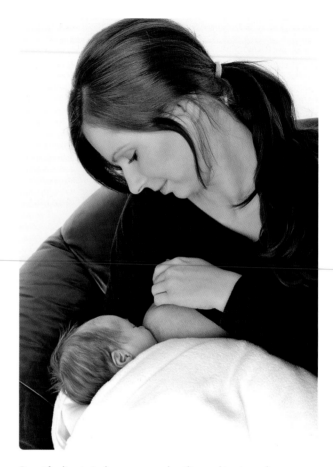

Breastfeeding isn't always as smooth sailing and instinctual as women are led to believe. Take a class before you deliver to learn the basics and consult with a lactation specialist in the event you have problems.

What to do if breastfeeding doesn't work well? Breastfeeding isn't always a smooth-sailing adventure. It's not always as instinctual as many women are led to believe. Sure, breastfeeding is the most natural way to feed your baby, but every baby and mother are unique, and there's a learning curve for each mother-baby couple.

Sign up for a breastfeeding class before you have your baby to learn how the process works, what the basic techniques are, and what to expect during the first days to weeks. If you have trouble after your baby is born and you're still in the hospital, ask your postpartum nurse for help. Most breastfeeding challenges can be solved with a few simple solutions, such as repositioning baby or adding pillows or blankets for support. If your nipples are painful, your nurse can help by providing special breast-friendly creams and bandages, helping you improve baby's latch, or if necessary, supplying a breast shield.

If you need more help than your postpartum nurse can offer, ask for a lactation consultant. These are custom-trained breastfeeding specialists who know all the tricks of the trade. They're breastfeeding miracle workers. Your hospital or birth center should have one on staff. You can also find private lactation consultants in most major cities, and they're usually covered by insurance.

What if you try everything and still can't breastfeed? Then consider pumping your milk and feeding it to your baby in a bottle. If that doesn't work for you, then be grateful you live in a country where formula is readily available. Though breast is best most of the time, sometimes formula and a bottle are the only way to go. Don't beat yourself up about this. Formula provides an excellent way to nourish your baby when breastfeeding just isn't happening. Choosing to use formula is not a judgment call, not a testament to your womanhood, or a statement about what kind of mother you are—it's food. Most babies do just fine with formula.

Discussing Your Plan with Your Health Care Provider and Your Partner/Labor Coach

Your birth plan can be a very effective tool for ensuring that you and your health care provider and/or labor support person have talked through the important details of your baby's birth and how they will be handled. Talking through the details ahead of time will give everyone the opportunity to resolve any issues up front, while there's still time to do so. For example, if you strongly disagree with a routine hospital procedure, discussing it ahead of time can give both you *and* your health care provider the opportunity to say why you feel strongly about something and what can—or can't—be done differently. (Remember: There may not be time to discuss such things once you're actually in labor.)

Also, if there are certain aspects of your birth plan that your health care provider does not believe would be safe for you and your baby, you'll have the opportunity to discuss that ahead of time. He or she may advise you to change certain aspects of your birth plan accordingly. (And if you have enough disagreements on your birth plan that you feel strongly about, perhaps you'll want to consider switching to a health care provider whose vision is more in line with your own.)

Inside Information

What do your labor nurse, midwife, and obstetrician really think of your birth plan? It depends on what it includes. Generally, we think they're a great idea. They show that mom has done her homework, knows what to expect, and is somewhat prepared for her labor and birth. She's put some thought into how she wants things to go and is assertive enough to make her wishes known. We love that.

But there are birth plans and then there are *birth plans*. Some go so far beyond what's reasonable or necessary, they're more like legal documents or blueprints than anything related to birth. Because every birth is a unique situation involving two different bodies, there's no way to know in advance exactly how birth will go and no guarantee the plans you've made are going to work out at all. Whenever possible, your providers aim to please. They try to make your birth plans come true, but keep in mind: babies never read those plans and often have a few ideas of their own about how birth's going to go. Hopefully you've chosen a health care provider whose general practice is in line with what you want so you don't have to second-guess him or her throughout your labor.

Any experienced labor nurse or provider knows the basics of what most mothers want even without seeing their birth plan. "Birth plan parents" generally want a low-intervention birth, though some are wide open to epidurals or other interventions. Your birth plan might have a list of things you do and don't want us to do and most of the time, we're more than happy to oblige. In fact, we probably would do them (or not) anyway, even if they weren't on your plan.

If a woman comes in with a very stringent plan dictating all kinds of guidelines she wants us to guarantee, no matter what, it indicates to staff that we have a patient who needs a lot of control, might be afraid of us and her own labor process, and is worried we're going to do stuff to her that will sabotage her birth experience. That's a challenging situation for all involved, especially if mom thinks her care providers are batting for the wrong team.

We do our best to help that frightened mother feel safe, respected, and well informed throughout her birth experience. Sometimes, however, when her labor doesn't go as planned, or if it was a longer, harder, and more painful experience than expected, she might feel traumatized, disappointed, and even hostile. For example, if she "caves in" and gets an epidural, when she was absolutely positive she'd go all natural, her harshest critic will undoubtedly be herself. That can really ding up her self-esteem. We wish she'd cut herself some slack in her birth plan and allowed herself some flexibility.

While we don't know of any studies to back this up, it does seem like the mothers who have the longest, most specific birth plans tend to have the most difficult births. The moms who come in with laminated three-pagers are the ones who wind up in the operating room with their baby in the NICU. The moms who come in with flexible plans that are more like wish lists than contracts are the ones who seem to have the smoothest time of it. Maybe that's because, as with all elements of parenting, flexibility is key.

Once you've reviewed your plan with your partner, labor support team, and health care provider and made any necessary adjustments, you'll want to print several copies. Give one to your health care provider to put in your chart. Give one to your labor coach. (You may even want to consider making a few important notes on this one, specifically for your labor coach, including instructions on how you'd like him or her to support you during labor, for example, "Please rub my back here" or "Please don't turn on the television to check the score on the game while I'm in labor!") Pack a few copies of your birth plan in your hospital bag, just in case you find yourself with a team of nurses or other health care providers who are unfamiliar with your preferences.

Some Sample Birth Plans

You can find plenty of great sample birth plans online. Before you begin writing your own, it's a good idea to look at a wide array of examples, from checklists, to bulleted lists, to paragraph-style plans. Be sure to read some real-world examples of other women's final birth plans, especially the ones who had a birth that sounds like one you'd like to have! Here are some good sources to get you started:

- Birthing Naturally's sample birth plans, www.birthingnaturally.net/birthplan/sample /index.html
- Doulas.org sample birth plan, www.doulas.org /samplebirthplan.html

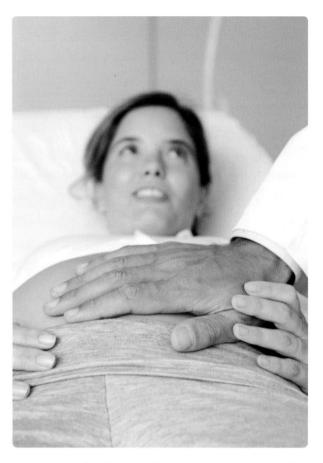

Do your homework and research all your options as you create a solid and realistic birth plan.

- BabyCenter.com's birth plan, http://assets.baby-center.com/ims/Content/birthplan_pdf.pdf
- The Bump's birth plan, http://pregnant .thebump.com/pregnancy/pregnancy-tools /articles/tool-birth-plan.aspx

Creating Your Own Birth Plan: A Birth Plan Template

Here's a template to get you started thinking about your own birth plan. It's by no means completely comprehensive, but it will give you a good overview of the types of things you might want to include in your own birth plan.

Name: ....

Due date: ....

MY LABOR SUPPORT TEAM:

I'd like the following people to be present for my baby's labor and delivery [include their names for the sake of your nurses and health care provider]:

....

....

....

....

....

THE THREE MOST IMPORTANT THINGS TO KEEP IN MIND ABOUT MY LABOR AND DELIVERY PREFERENCES ARE:

1. ....

....

....

2. ....

....

....

3. ....

....

....

PLEASE NOTE THAT I HAVE THE FOLLOWING MEDICAL CONDITIONS:

1. ....

....

....

2. ....

....

....

3. ....

....

....

[Be sure to note whether you tested positive for group B strep, gestational diabetes, an Rh incompatibility, etc.]

MY BABY'S BIRTH IS PLANNED AS A(N):

☐ unmedicated, vaginal birth at home

☐ unmedicated, vaginal birth at a birth center

☐ unmedicated, vaginal birth at a hospital

☐ vaginal birth in a hospital, with an epidural

☐ induction of labor in a hospital

☐ vaginal birth after Cesarean

☐ planned Cesarean

ENVIRONMENT:

I'd like to:

☐ Dim the lights

☐ Play music

☐ Wear my own clothing

☐ Be able to move around throughout my labor and delivery

☐ Eat and drink as needed

☐ Have the room as quiet as possible

☐ Other: ....
....
....

Comments/notes: ....
....
....
....
....
....
....
....
....
....
....
....
....

ABOUT ROUTINE HOSPITAL PROCEDURES AND/OR INTERVENTIONS:

As long as my baby and I are doing fine, I would prefer to:

☐ have intermittent rather than continuous fetal monitoring

☐ hydrate myself by drinking fluids rather than having an IV

☐ wear my own clothing

☐ be able to move around throughout my labor

☐ have my partner and/or labor coach with me at all times

☐ allow my labor to happen and progress naturally, without imposing any strict timelines or interventions unless absolutely necessary

☐ have minimal vaginal exams

☐ not have my membranes stripped or water broken unless it is absolutely medically necessary

☐ not have my labor induced with Pitocin unless it is absolutely medically necessary

☐ not have an episiotomy unless it is absolutely medically necessary

☐ not have my baby's birth assisted by forceps or vacuum extraction unless it is absolutely medically necessary

Comments/notes: ....
....
....
....
....
....
....
....
....
....
....
....
....

MANAGING THE PAIN OF LABOR:

I'd like to use the following tools and techniques to help manage the pain of labor and the delivery of my baby:

☐ Breathing techniques

☐ Meditation

☐ Hypnosis

☐ Massage

☐ Imagery and visualization

☐ Cold or warm compresses

☐ Movement and various labor positions

☐ A warm tub or shower

☐ A birthing ball

☐ A birthing stool

☐ Opiates/narcotics

☐ An epidural

☐ Please do not offer me pain medication; I'll request it if needed.

Comments/notes: ....
....
....
....
....
....
....
....
....
....
....
....

DELIVERING THE BABY:

☐ I'd like to push as my body directs me to.

☐ I prefer having someone coach me through pushing.

☐ I'd like to watch my baby being born in a mirror.

☐ I'd like to be able to touch my baby as she is crowning and being born.

☐ I prefer to have my partner help "catch" the baby.

☐ I prefer for my partner to stay near my head during the delivery.

☐ I'd like to have my partner cut the cord.

☐ I'd like to have my baby placed in my arms or on my chest immediately after birth.

☐ I'd like to have my baby cleaned up and assessed before I hold him or her.

I'd like to try these positions for giving birth:

☐ All fours

☐ Leaning or kneeling

☐ Lunging

☐ Squatting

☐ Lying on my side

☐ Semi-reclining

☐ Other: ....
....
....

If I need a C-section:

☐ I would like to have time to discuss with my partner, if time permits.

☐ I would like my partner to be present at all times, if possible.

☐ I would like to remain conscious, if possible.

☐ I would like to have the screen lowered so that I can see my baby being born.

☐ I would like to see and/or hold my baby as soon as possible.

☐ I would like my partner to remain with the baby at all times.

AFTER THE DELIVERY:

☐ I'd like to have a sample of my baby's cord blood collected

    ☐ for a private bank

    ☐ for a public bank (not available in all states)

☐ I'd prefer not to be given Pitocin when delivering the placenta unless it's absolutely necessary.

☐ I'd like to keep the baby with me at all times, including for any newborn procedures.

☐ I'd like my partner to accompany the baby for any newborn procedures.

☐ I would like to postpone any newborn procedures until I have had a chance to bond with my baby (at least forty-five minutes to one hour).

☐ I'd like to try breastfeeding as soon as possible.

☐ I plan to formula feed my baby.

☐ I plan to try a combination of formula feeding and breastfeeding.

☐ I would like to have my baby boy circumcised.

☐ I do not want my baby boy to be circumcised.

☐ I will decide about circumcision at a later date.

☐ I would like to stay at the hospital for as long as possible.

☐ I would like to return home as soon as possible.

☐ Other: ....

....

....

I do not want my baby to have:

☐ a bath; I would like to give my baby his first bath

☐ vitamin K; I will sign a waiver if need be

☐ antibiotic eye ointments; I will sign a waiver if need be

☐ any vaccinations or injections of any kind without my prior written consent

☐ sugar water

☐ formula

☐ a pacifier

APPENDIX

A Tri-by-Tri Guide:
A week-by-week checklist for each trimester
and a timeline to prepare for your birth experience

	What's Happening	*Preparing for Your Baby's Birth*
Week 1	Although you're not actually pregnant, week one marks the start of 40 weeks of pregnancy, with the start of your menstrual cycle. For women with regular, 28-day cycles, the most fertile times to conceive are generally around 14 days after your period starts.	Even though you haven't yet conceived your baby, now is a great time to think through your own birthing style and begin to research the best health care provider for you. It's a good idea to have a checkup with your health care provider before you decide to conceive.
Week 2	Your ovaries are getting ready to release the egg that, once it meets some lucky sperm, will become the fertilized egg that grows into your beautiful baby.	If you're not already, you should be taking a prenatal vitamin. (It's recommended that you start taking them 3 months prior to conception, so the sooner the better.) You can find plenty of great over-the-counter options from which to choose—the generic vitamins are much cheaper and very similar to prescription vitamins.
Week 3	If you're going to conceive, this may be the week when sperm meets egg, and your journey officially begins!	If you haven't already researched and selected a health care provider and the place where you'd like to deliver, you'll want to do so soon. See chapter 1 for information on finding the right fit for you.
Week 4	By the end of this week, a home pregnancy test will usually be able to tell you that you're pregnant. Congratulations!	Be sure to contact your health care provider to find out when he or she would like to see you for your first prenatal appointment. This generally happens between 8 and 10 weeks after your last menstrual period.

	What's Happening	*Preparing for Your Baby's Birth*
Week 5	Your baby's heart is beginning to pump blood, organs are beginning to develop, and arm and leg buds are appearing.	Now may be a good time to start thinking about what type of childbirth education classes you'd like to take. See chapter 1 for an overview of several birthing schools of thought.
Week 6	Your baby is about a quarter of an inch (6 mm) long now, and her nose, mouth, and ears are beginning to form.	Have you started thinking about who will be part of your labor team?
Week 7	If you haven't already, you may be experiencing some of the "joys" of pregnancy, like nausea, food aversions, frequent urination, and extreme exhaustion.	Get ready for your first prenatal appointment by reading the chapter that most closely aligns with your own birthing style. You may also want to skim through this book's advice on birth plans so you can get a sense of the topics you may want to talk through with your health care provider.
Week 8	Your baby's "tail" (the precursor to your baby's growing spine) is just about gone now, making him look a lot less like a reptile and a lot more like a baby!	If you have your first prenatal appointment this week, pay close attention to the rapport you have with your health care provider, the office staff, and facilities where you'll be spending a lot of time for the next few months. If it doesn't feel right, it's not too late to find a health care provider that feels like a better fit for you. Now's also a good time to discuss any first-trimester screening tests that your health care provider recommends.
Week 9	By now, an ultrasound or Doppler device may be able to detect your baby's heartbeat.	Have you spoken with your partner about your own hopes, wishes, and plans for baby's birth? It's a great time to begin aligning your vision and building your support network. Around 11 to 13 weeks, your health care provider may offer a "nuchal translucency" ultrasound to screen for the chromosomal disorders Down Syndrome and Trisomy 18.

	What's Happening	*Preparing for Your Baby's Birth*
Week 10	Your baby is now officially a fetus, measuring about an inch (2.5 cm) long.	Have you signed up for a childbirth education class? See chapter 1 for an overview. Sign up early, as many classes book up weeks in advance.
Week 11	Your baby is looking much more human now, with hands, feet, fingers, toes, ears, a nose, and more features beginning to take shape. Your baby is about 3 inches (7.5 cm) long now, and weighs about an ounce (28 g).	Why not take advantage of these early weeks of pregnancy to practice some relaxation, meditation, and visualization techniques for managing the pain of labor? See chapter 10 for some tips and techniques.

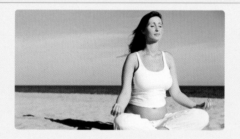

Week 12	You may be starting to have more energy and less nausea at this point. This week, your baby's beginning to develop reflexes such as flexing his fingers and toes and making sucking motions with his mouth. Your baby's brain is developing rapidly.	With your health care provider's approval, why not make use of your newfound energy to try a prenatal yoga class? It'll give you the opportunity to practice some of the squats, lunges, and other labor positions detailed in chapter 10.
Week 13	Your health care provider may suggest that you have a test called a quad screen anywhere between 15 and 18 weeks to test for neural tube defects, Down Syndrome, and other genetic disorders. (If you already had the nuchal translucency test, then you'll only have an alpha-fetoprotein [AFP] test drawn around 16 weeks to screen for neural tube defects.)	Now is a good time to think about whether you'd like to hire a doula to assist you during your labor.

	What's Happening	Preparing for Your Baby's Birth
Week 14	This is the start of your second trimester, the "honeymoon trimester," when women tend to feel their best and the rate of miscarriage drops dramatically.	During your second trimester, you'll most likely be seeing your health care provider every 4 weeks. Consider bringing your partner or labor coach to several appointments, so he or she can also get to know your health care provider before your baby's birth.
Week 15	You may be starting to feel Braxton Hicks contractions in the coming weeks. They're your uterus's way of practicing for the real contractions that will start dilating your cervix during labor.	Have you shared your birth plan with your partner and health care provider? See chapter 11 for tips and sample birth plans.
Week 16	If you haven't already had an ultrasound, your health care provider will probably recommend doing one between 18 and 20 weeks to assess your baby's development.	Even though you may be envisioning your baby's "perfect birth," labor and delivery can be unpredictable. Be sure to read through chapter 9 on unplanned Cesarean delivery, so you won't be caught off guard if you or your baby should need a lifesaving surgery.
Week 17	You may be starting to feel the baby move between now and 22 weeks (or sooner if it's not your first pregnancy).	Have you thought about the support systems you'll need in place after the birth?
Week 18	Your baby now measures about 5½ inches (14 cm) long and weighs about 5 ounces (142 g).	If you'd like to find out the sex of your baby, your health care provider or ultrasound technician should be able to tell whether your baby is a boy or girl via an ultrasound.
Week 19	Research has shown that your baby may be able to hear your voice by now.	You'll want to begin taking childbirth classes over the course of the next few weeks.

	What's Happening	Preparing for Your Baby's Birth
Week 32	By now your baby weighs almost 4 pounds (1.4 kg) and measures almost 16-inches (41 cm)-long.	Now would be a great time to review the stages of labor in chapter 10, so you'll know what to expect once labor begins.
Week 33	Right about now, you may be feeling a strong urge to "nest." (It's nature's way of getting you ready to care for a baby, and has been attributed to a surge in adrenaline.)	Take advantage of the energy you're feeling now to practice your labor positions.
Week 34	Your baby is building fatty tissue to help regulate his body temperature after birth. His central nervous system and lungs are maturing more every day.	You may want to consider taking an infant CPR class now, because it will be harder to do so once you have a newborn to take care of.
Week 35	Your health care provider may want to test you between 35 and 37 weeks for group B streptococcus bacteria, which can infect the baby at birth and make her ill if it is left untreated.	If you test positive for group B strep, your health care provider will speak with you about getting to the hospital early in your labor to begin a course of IV antibiotics to protect your baby during the delivery.
Week 36	If he or she hasn't already, your baby is now moving into position for delivery.	At 36 weeks, you'll most likely start seeing your health care provider every week until your baby's born.
Week 37	If your baby is not in a head-down position, your health care provider may recommend a procedure called external cephalic version, where she'll try to move your baby into position by placing her hands on your belly and pushing.	It's time to start packing your hospital bag with all of the items you'd like to help manage the pain of delivery. (See chapter 10 for ideas.)

	What's Happening	*Preparing for Your Baby's Birth*
Week 38	Your pregnancy is now officially considered "full term." If your baby were born at this point, she would have more than a 99 percent chance of being born perfectly healthy. But most health care practitioners agree that it's best to keep that bun in the oven until spontaneous labor begins.	Your health care provider has no doubt discussed with you what you should do if you notice a "bloody show," if you begin having strong and regular contractions, or if your water breaks.
Week 39	If you have a planned Cesarean, your health care provider may want to deliver your baby soon.	If you have a scheduled Cesarean, review chapter 8, so you'll know what to expect.
Week 40	You've reached your due date! You could be meeting your baby any time now.	Now's a great time to review the chapter that's most closely aligned to your own birth plan (and, of course, chapter 9 on unplanned Cesareans, so you won't be caught off guard should you need one).
Week 41	Still pregnant? Remember: Due dates are an approximation, and try not to get too hung up on the fact that you're now "overdue." Try to get some rest for the marathon of labor, delivery, and newborn days ahead.	If you've gone past your due date, your health care provider may want to see you twice a week for ultrasounds and fetal monitoring to make sure that you and baby are doing well.
Week 42	Still pregnant? You're no doubt getting frustrated by now. Hang in there and focus on the fact that you're going to meet your baby soon!	Though some midwives and birth centers will allow women to go beyond 42 weeks before inducing labor, your health care provider may decide that it's time to induce you if you haven't gone into labor naturally by now.

REFERENCES

CHAPTER 1

www.hypnobirthing.com.

http://health.howstuffworks.com/pregnancy-and-parenting/pregnancy/labor-delivery/hypnobirthing.htm.

www.bradleybirth.com/.

www.bradleybirth.com/WhyBradley.aspx.

www.lamaze.org/WhoWeAre/AboutLamaze/tabid/105/Default.aspx.

www.lamaze.org/AboutLamaze/MissionandVision/LamazePhilosophyofBirth/tabid/378/Default.aspx.

www.lamaze.org/Default.aspx?tabid=90.

www.birthingfromwithin.com/mission.

www.birthingfromwithin.com/philosophy.

www.ChildbirthConnection.org

Accreditation Commission for Midwifery Education

North American Registry of Midwives

American College of Nurse Midwives

American Association of Naturopathic Physicians

American Association of Naturopathic Midwives

The American College of Naturopathic Obstetrics

CHAPTER 2

"Homebirth, Know the Pros and Cons," Mayo Cinic, June 21, 2011, www.mayoclinic.com/health/home-birth/MY01713.

American Pregnancy Association, www.americanpregnancy.org/labornbirth/homebirth.html.

ACOG Opinion on Planned Home Birth, www.acog.org/from_home/publications/press_releases/nr01-20-11.cfm.

Tina Cassidy, *Birth* (New York: Atlantic Monthly Press, 2006), 54–55.

Debora Boucher, Catherine Bennett, Barbara McFarlin, and Rixa Freeze, "Staying Home to Give Birth: Why Women in the United States Choose Home Birth," *Journal of Midwifery & Women's Health* 54, No. 2 (2009): 119–26.

American College of Nurse-Midwives, "Home Births," *Position Statement* (Washington, DC: American College of Nurse-Midwives, 2005), http://midwife.org/siteFiles/position/home-Birth.pdf.

Ackermann-Liebrich et al., "Home versus Hospital Deliveries: Follow-up Study of Matched Pairs for Procedures and Outcome," Zurich Study Team, *BMJ* 313 (1996): 1313–18, Pub Med (PMID 8942694).

"New Figures from the Netherlands on the Safety of Home Births," published on 04/15/09 by A. de Jonge et al., "Perinatal Mortality and Morbidity in a Nationwide Cohort of 529,688 Low-Risk Planned Home and Hospital Births," *BJOG* (2009), doi: 10.1111/j.1471-0528.2009.0217.

Marian F. MacDorman, Fay Menacker, and Eugene Declercq, "Trends and Characteristics of Home and Other Out-of-Hospital Births in the United States, 1990–2006," *CDC National Vital Statistics Report* 58, No. 11 (revised August 30, 2010), www.cdc.gov/nchs/data/nvsr/nvsr58/nvsr58_11.PDF.

H. C. Woodcock et al., "A Matched Cohort Study of Planned Home and Hospital Births in Western Australia 1981–1987," *Midwifery* 10, No. 3 (1994): 125–35, Pub Med (PMID 7639843), www.ncbi.nlm.nih.gov/pubmed/7639843;

P. A. Janssen et al., "Outcomes of Planned Home Births versus Planned Hospital Births after Regulation of Midwifery in British Columbia," *CMAJ* 166, No. 3 (2002): 315–23, Pub Med Central (PMC 99310), www.ncbi.nlm.nih.gov/pmc/articles/PMC99310/.

Eryn Brown, "Birth: U.S. Home Births Increase 20% from 2004 to 2008," *Los Angeles Times*, May 20, 2011, http://articles.latimes.com/2011/may/20/news/la-heb-home-births-increase-20110520.

Centers for Disease Control and Prevention, "Home and Other Out-of-Hospital Births," *National Vital Statistics Report* 58, No. 11 (revised August 30, 2010), www.cdc.gov/nchs/data/nvsr/nvsr58/nvsr58_11.PDF.

Elizabeth R. Cluett and Ethel Burns, "Immersion in Water in Labour and Birth," ed. Cochrane Pregnancy and Childbirth Group (John Wiley and Sons, April 15, 2009, assessed as up-to-date, August 23, 2011), The Cochrane Library, doi: 10.1002/14651858.CD000111.pub3.

Catherine Elton, "Should American Women Learn to Give Birth at Home?" *Time*, September 4, 2010, www.time.com/time/magazine/article/0,9171,2011940,00.html.

Royal College of Obstetricians and Gynaecologists and Royal College of Midwives, "Home Births." *Joint Statement No 2.* (London, England: RCOG and Royal College of Midwives, April 2007), www.rcog.org.uk/womens-health/clinical-guidance/home-births.

World Health Organization, *Care in Normal Birth: A Practical Guide* (Geneva, Switzerland: Department of Reproductive Health and Research, World Health Organization, 1996), accessed September 14, 2009, http://whqlibdoc.who.int/hq/1996/WHO_FRH_MSM_96.24.pdf.

New Zealand Health Information Service, *Report on Maternity: Maternal and Newborn Information* (Wellington, New Zealand: New Zealand Ministry of Health, 2007), accessed September 14, 2009, www.nzhis.govt.nz/moh.nsf/pagesns/73/$File/maternityreport04.pdf.

J. A. Martin et al., "Births: Final Data for 2005," CDC *National Vital Statistics Report* 56, No. 6 (December 5, 2007), www.cdc.gov/nchs/data/nvsr/nvsr56/nvsr56_06.pdf.

National Collaborating Centre for Women's and Children's Health, Commissioned by the National Institute for Health and Clinical Excellence, *Intrapartum Care: Care of Healthy Women and Their Babies during Childbirth* (London, England: Royal College of Obstetricians and Gynaecologists, March 22, 2007), www.nice.org.uk/nicemedia/pdf/IPC-cons-fullguideline.pdf.

Committee on Obstetric Practice, "Planned Home Birth," *Committee Opinion*, No. 476 (American College of Obstetricians and Gynecologists, February 2011).

"Does Home Birth Empower Women, or Imperil Them *and* Their Babies?" *OBG Management* 21, No. 8 (August 2009), www.obgmanagement.com/article_pages.asp?AID=7776#bib11.

American Public Health Association, "Increasing Access to Out-of-Hospital Maternity Care Services through State-Regulated and Nationally-Certified Direct-Entry Midwives," *APHA Policy Statement #20013* (January 1, 2001).

National Birthday Trust Fund, *Research Summaries: Report of the Confidential Enquiry into Home Births*, ed. G. Chamberlain, A. Wraight, and P. Crowley, Home Birth.org, www.homebirth.org.uk/homebirth2.htm.

"Resource A–Z," Childbirth Connection, www.childbirthconnection.org/article.asp?ck=10159.

A.D.A.M. Medical Encyclopedia, s.v. "HELLP syndrome," Pub Med Health, www.ncbi.nlm.nih.gov/pubmedhealth/PMH0001892/.

A.D.A.M. Medical Encyclopedia, s.v. "APGAR," Pub Med Health, www.ncbi.nlm.nih.gov/pubmedhealth/PMH0003880/.

CHAPTER 3

American Association of Birth Centers, www.birthcenters.org/birth-center-faq/bc-difference.php.

American Association of Birth Centers, www.birthcenters.org/birth-center-faq/what-people-say.php.

Kim Schworm Acousta, "The Vanishing Birth Center" *Fit Pregnancy*, Dec/Jan 2010, www.fitpregnancy.com/unsorted/vanishing-birth-center.

J. A. Martin et al., "Births: Final Data for 2004," *National Vital Statistics Report* 55, No. 1 (2006): 1–101.

American Congress of Obstetricians and Gynecologists, "ACOG Committee Opinion No. 476: Planned Home Birth," abstract, *Obstetrics & Gynecology* 117, No. 2 (February 2011): 425–28.

Midwives Alliance of North America, from American Academy of Pediatrics and American Congress of Obstetricians and Gynecologists, *Guidelines for Perinatal Care*, 5th ed. (Elk Grove Village, IL: AAP/ACOG, 2002), http://mana.org/ACOGStatement.html.

Katherine Shaver, "Birth Centers' Closures Limit Delivery Options," *The Washington Post*, May 18, 2007, www.washingtonpost.com/wp-dyn/content/article/2007/05/17AR2007051702301.html.

"Birth Center: An Option for Pregnancy Care," Mayo Clinic. com, October 12, 2010, www.mayoclinic.com/health/ birth-center/MY01258.

The American College of Nurse Midwives

American Nurses Association

Birth Network National

Citizens for Midwifery

Coalition for Improving Maternity Services

Lamaze International

White Ribbon Alliance for Safe Motherhood

CHAPTER 4

Joyce A. Martin et al., "Final Data for 2009," *CDC National Vital Statistics Report* 60, No. 1 (November 2011).

Eugene R. Declercq, Carol Sakala, Maureen P. Corry, and Sandra Applebaum, *Listening to Mothers II: Report of the Second National U.S. Survey of Women's Childbearing Experiences* (New York, NY: Childbirth Connection, 2006).

OB Laborist.org, www.oblaborist.org/patient.php.

David Legrew, "Strategies for Reducing Unnecessary Cesarean Section," *American Journal of Obstetrics & Gynecology* 178, No. 6 (June 1998), 1207–14.

Brady E. Hamilton, Joyce A. Martin, and Stephanie J. Ventura, "Births: Preliminary Data for 2010," *CDC National Vital Statistics Report* 60, No. 2 (November 2011): 6, www.cdc.gov/ nchs/data/nvsr/nvsr60/nvsr60_02.pdf.

DONA International, www.dona.org/.

Elizabeth G. Baxley and Robert W. Gobbo, "Shoulder Dystocia," *American Family Physician* 69, No. 7 (April 1, 2004): 1707–14.

CHAPTER 5

Committee on Obstetric Practice, American Society of Anesthesiologists, "Pain Relief During Labor," *Committee Opinion,* No. 295 (American Congress of Obstetricians and Gynecologists, July 2004, replaces No. 231, February 2000, reaffirmed 2008), www.acog.org/Resources_And_Publications/ Committee_Opinions/Committee_on_Obstetric_Practice/ Pain_Relief_During_Labor.aspx.

Linda J. Smith, "Impact of Birthing Practices on Breastfeeding," Dyad, *Journal of Midwifery & Women's Health* 52, No. 6 (Nov/ Dec 2007): 621–30.

"Epidural Anesthesia," American Pregnancy Association, last updated August 2007, www.americanpregnancy.org/laborn-birth/epidural.html.

"Epidural versus Non-Epidural or No Analgesia in Labour," Anim-Somuah M., Smyth RMD, Jones, The Cochrane Collaboration, December 7, 2011 http://summaries.cochrane. org/CD000331/epidurals-for-pain-relief-in-labour.

Hemant K. Satpathy, "Labor and Delivery, Analgesia, Regional and Local," in *EMedicine Medscape Reference,* ed. Alex Macario, updated May 9, 2011, http://emedicine.medscape. com/article/149337-overview#a15.

Marjorie Greenfield, "Epidural - Pros, Cons and Considerations: Natural Childbirth versus Epidural," *Birth Buddies* (blog), April 22, 2007, http://birthbuddy.wordpress.com/2007/04/22/ epidural-pros-cons-considerations/.

Samantha Phillips, "Epidurals: Fact vs. Fiction," *Fit Pregnancy,* April/May 2010, www.fitpregnancy.com/yourpregnancy/ labor_delivery/epidural-facts-combined-spinal-epidural-csec-tions-92115779.html.

"Combined Spinal-Epidural (CSE) for Labor Analgesia: The Walking Epidural," Anesthesiology Info.com, 2005, http://an-esthesiologyinfo.com/articles/09152002.php.

"Using Narcotics for Pain Relief During Childbirth," The American Pregnancy Association, www.americanpregnancy. org/labornbirth/narcotics.html.

"Labor Epidurals and Childbirth Education Classes," Anesthesiology Info.com, 2005, http://anesthesiologyinfo. com/articles/07162002b.php.

Committee on Obstetric Practice, "Pain Relief during Labor," July 2004.

CHAPTER 6

Deborah B. Ehrenthal, Xiaozhang Jiang, and Donna M. Strobino, "Labor Induction and the Risk of a Cesarean Delivery Among Nulliparous Women at Term," *Obstetrics & Gynecology* 116, No. 1 (July 2010): 35–42, http://journals.lww.com/greenjournal/Fulltext/2010/07000/Labor_Induction_and_the_Risk_of_a_Cesarean.8.aspx.

"Induction in Labor," Mayo Clinic.com, July 22, 2011, www.mayoclinic.com/health/labor-induction/MY00642.

J. Kavanagh, A. J. Kelly, and J. Thomas, "Breast Stimulation for Cervical Ripening and Induction of Labour," *Cochrane Database System Review* 3 (July 20, 2005), The Cochrane Database (CD003392).

Jonathan Schaffir et al., "Sexual Intercourse at Term Does Not Hasten the Onset of Labor or Result in Cervical Ripening," *Obstetrics & Gynecology* 107 (2006): 1310–14.

Peng Chiong Tan, Anggeriana Andi, Noor Azmi, and M. N. Noraihan, "Effect of Coitus at Term on Length of Gestation, Induction of Labor, and Mode of Delivery," *Obstetrics & Gynecology* 108, No. 1 (July 2006): 134–40.

"Natural Herbs and Vitamins during Pregnancy," American Pregnancy Association, www.americanpregnancy.org/pregnancyhealth/naturalherbsvitamins.html.

Natural Medicines Database, www.naturaldatabase.com.

Josie L. Tenore, "Methods for Cervical Ripening and Induction of Labor, *American Family Physician* 67, No. 10 (May 15, 2003): 2123–28, www.aafp.org/afp/2003/0515/p2123.html.

"Less than 39 Weeks Toolkit," March of Dimes, www.marchofdimes.com/professionals/medicalresources_39weeks.html.

American Congress of Obstetricians and Gynecology, "Induction of Labor," *ACOG Practice Bulletin*, No. 107 (Washington, DC: American Congress of Obstetricians and Gynecology, August 2009).

"Inducing Labor," American Pregnancy Association, www.americanpregnancy.org/labornbirth/inducinglabor.html.

CHAPTER 7

"Cesarean Section: Why Is the National U.S. Cesarean Section Rate So High?" Childbirth Connection, updated May 17, 2012, www.childbirthconnection.org/article.asp?ck=10456.

"Vaginal Birth After Cesarean: New Insights," Paper presented at NIH Consensus Development Conference, Bethesda, Maryland, March 8-10, 2010, http://consensus.nih.gov/2010/vbacabstracts.htm.

"QuickStats: Total and Primary Cesarean Rate and Vaginal Birth after Previous Cesarean (VBAC) Rate, United States, 1989–2003," Centers for Disease Control and Prevention, www.cdc.gov/mmwr/preview/mmwrhtml/mm5402a5.htm.

M. J. McMahon, E. R. Luther, W. A. Bowes, and A. F. Olshan, "Comparison of a Trial of Labor with an Elective Second Cesarean Section," *New England Journal of Medicine* 335 (1996): 689–95.

M. Lydon-Rochelle, V. L. Holt, T. R. Easterling, and D. P. Martin, "Risk of Uterine Rupture during Labor Among Women with Prior Cesarean Delivery," *New England Journal of Medicine* 345 (2001): 3-8.

American Congress of Obstetricians and Gynecologists, "Vaginal Birth after Previous Cesarean Delivery," *ACOG Practice Bulletin*, No. 54 (Washington, DC: American Congress of Obstetricians and Gynecologists, July 10, 2004).

American Congress of Obstetricians and Gynecologists, "Vaginal Birth after Previous Cesarean Delivery," *ACOG Practice Bulletin*, No. 115 (Washington, DC: American Congress of Obstetricians and Gynecologists, August 2010).

Tekoa L. King, "First Do No Harm: The Case for Vaginal Birth after Cesarean," *Journal of Midwifery & Women's Health* 55, No. 3 (May–June 2010): 202–5, article first published online, December 24, 2010, American College of Nurse Midwives, doi: 10.1016/j.jmwh.2010.03.010.

"Best Evidence: VBAC or Repeat C-Section," Childbirth Connection, www.childbirthconnection.org/article.asp?ck=10210.

American College of Nurse-Midwives, "Care for Women Desiring Vaginal Birth after Cesarean," *Journal of Midwifery & Women's Health* 56, No. 5 (September/October 2011): 517–25, article first published online, August 25, 2011, http://onlinelibrary.wiley.com/doi/10.1111/j.1542-2011.2011.00112.x/full.

"VBAC (vaginal birth after C-section)," Mayo Clinic.com, www.mayoclinic.com/health/vbac/MY01143/DSECTION=how-you-prepare.

John T. Queenan, "How to Stop the Relentless Rise in Cesarean Deliveries," editorial, *Obstetrics & Gynecology* 118, No. 2 (August 2011), quoted from VBAC.com.

James R. Scott, "Vaginal Birth after Cesarean: A Common-Sense Approach," Abstract, *Obstetrics & Gynecology*, 118, No. 2 (August 2011), http://journals.lww.com/greenjournal/Abstract/2011/08000/Vaginal_Birth_After_Cesarean_Delivery__A.21.aspx.

CHAPTER 8

Chaya Merrill and Claudia Steiner, "Hospitalizations Related to Childbirth, 2003, *H-CUP Statistical Brief #11* (Rockville, MD: Agency for Healthcare Research and Quality, June 2008), www.hcup-us.ahrq.gov/reports/statbriefs/sb11.jsp.

"Cesarean Birth FAQ," American Congress of Obstetricians and Gynecologists, May 2011, www.acog.org/~/media/For%20Patients/faq006.ashx?dmc=1&ts=20120119T2107159204.

Fay Menacker and Brady E. Hamilton, "Recent Trends in Cesarean Delivery in the United States," *National Center for Health Statistics Data Brief*, No. 35 (Centers for Disease Control and Prevention, March 2010).

Luz Gibbons et al., "The Global Numbers and Costs of Additionally Needed and Unnecessary Caesarean Sections Performed per Year: Overuse as a Barrier to Universal Coverage," *2010 World Health Report*, Background Paper 30 (World Health Organization, 2010), table 3, www.who.int/healthsystems/topics/financing/healthreport/30C-section-costs.pdf.

Brady E. Hamilton, Joyce A. Martin, and Stephanie J. Ventura, "Births: Preliminary Data for 2010," *CDC National Vital Statics Report* 60, No. 2 (November 2011).

Tekoa L. King, "First Do No Harm: The Case for Vaginal Birth after Cesarean," *Journal of Midwifery & Women's Health* 55, No. 3 (May–June 2010): 202–05, doi: 10.1016/j.jmwh.2010.03.010, article first published online, December 24, 2010.

Committee on Obstetric Practice, "Cesarean Delivery on Maternal Request," *Committee Opinion*, No. 394 (American Congress of Obstetricians and Gynecologists, December 2007, replaces No. 386, November 2007, reaffirmed 2010),

www.acog.org/Resources_And_Publications/Committee_Opinions/Committee_on_Obstetric_Practice/Cesarean_Delivery_on_Maternal_Request.

James Lumalcuri, and Ralph W. Hale, "Medical Liability an Ongoing Nemesis," *Obstetrics & Gynecology* 115, No. 2 (February 2010), table 3.

M. C. Tollånes, D. Moster, A. K. Daltveit, and L. M. Irgens, "Cesarean Section and Risk of Severe Childhood Asthma: A Population-Based Cohort Study," *Pediatrics* 53, No. 1 (July 2008): 112–16, Pub Med (PMID 18571547), www.ncbi.nlm.nih.gov/pubmed/18571547.

"C-Section: Medical Reasons," March of Dimes, www.marchof dimes.com/pregnancy/csection_indepth.html.

Helena A. Goldani et al., "Cesarean Delivery Is Associated with an Increased Risk of Obesity in Adulthood in a Brazilian Birth Cohort Study," *American Journal of Clinical Nutrition* 93, No. 6 (April 2011): 1344–47, Pub Med (PMID 21508088), www.ncbi.nlm.nih.gov/pubmed/21508088.

C. Roduit et al., "Asthma at 8 Years of Age in Children Born by Caesarean Section." *Thorax* 64, No. 2 (February 2009):107–13, Epub December 3, 2008.

For a comprehensive list of more related studies, see: http://electivecesarean.blogspot.com/2008/07/cesarean-asthma-link-is-only-one-of.html.

CHAPTER 9

"Cesarean Section: Rates for Total Cesarean Section, Primary Cesarean Section and Vaginal Birth after Cesarean Section (VBAC), United States, 1989–2010," Childbirth Connection, updated May 18, 2012, www.childbirthconnection.org/article.asp?ck=10554.

Michelle J. K. Osteman, Joyce A. Martin, T. J. Matthews, and Brady E. Hamilton, "Primary Cesarean and Vaginal Birth after Cesarean Delivery, by Race and Hispanic Origin of Mother: 27 States and Puerto Rico, 2008," table I-5, *CDC National Vital Statistics Reports* 59, No. 7 (July 27, 2011), www.cdc.gov/nchs/data/nvsr/nvsr59/nvsr59_07_tables.pdf.

"QuickStats: Total and Primary Cesarean Rate and Vaginal Birth after Previous Cesarean (VBAC) – United States 1989-2003," National Center for Health Statistics, National Vital Statistics System, annual files, 1989–2003, www.cdc.gov/mmwr/preview/mmwrhtml/mm5402a5.htm.

D. S. Gifford et al., "Lack of Progress in Labor as a Reason for Cesarean," *Obstetrics & Gynecology* 95, No. 4 (April 2000): 589–95, Pub Med (PMID 10725495), www.ncbi.nlm.nih.gov/pubmed/10725495.

"How to Cope If You Feel Disappointed after a Cesarean," Review of comment string, Baby Centre, LLC, www.babycentre.co.uk/pregnancy/labourandbirth/labourcomplications/disappointedaftercaesarean/.

"Unplanned Cesarean Deliveries Mar Mothers' Experience of Childbirth," American Psychological Association, www.apa.org/monitor/mar00/cesarean.aspx.

Marian F. MacDorman, Fay Menacker, and Eugene Declercq, "Cesarean Birth in the United States: Epidemiology, Trends, and Outcomes," *Clinics in Perinatology* 35(2008): 293–307, www2.cfpc.ca/local/user/files/%7BCB26B78C-E421-4510-A76E-BA338489A90D%7D/CS%20US%20Meneker%20%20and%20Declerque.pdf.

"Cesarean Section: Topic Overview," Web MD, www.webmd.com/baby/tc/cesarean-section-topic-overview.

Fay Menacker and Brady E. Hamilton, "Recent Trends in Cesarean Delivery in the United States," *NCHS Data Brief*, No. 35 (National Center for Health Statistics, March 2010), www.cdc.gov/nchs/data/databriefs/db35.pdf.

CHAPTER 10

Samantha Phillips, "Epidurals: Fact vs. Fiction," *Fit Pregnancy*, April/May, 2010, www.fitpregnancy.com/yourpregnancy/labor_delivery/epidural-facts-combined-spinal-epidural-csections-92115779.html.

"Stages of Labor: Baby, It's Time!" Mayo Clinic.com, www.mayoclinic.com/health/stages-of-labor/PR00106.

"Stages of Labor," March of Dimes, www.marchofdimes.com/pregnancy/vaginalbirth_indepth.html.

"The Stages of Labor," Baby Center, www.babycenter.com/stages-of-labor.

"The Rice Sock for Labor," *Birthing Naturally*, www.birthingnaturally.net/cn/tool/sock.html.

"Mind Over Matter," *Fit Pregnancy*, www.fitpregnancy.com/yourpregnancy/labor_delivery/mind-over-matter-40727857.html.

Wikipedia, s.v. "Hypnosis for labor," http://en.wikipedia.org/wiki/Hypnotherapy_in_childbirth.

VisualizingBirth.org, http://visualizingbirth.org/pages/introduction.

Gentlebirth.org, www.gentlebirth.org/archives/hypnosis.html#Affirmations.

Birth Buddies: Birthing without Fear, http://birthbuddy.wordpress.com/.

James Goodlatte and Kimberly Nelli, "Mental Imagery and Pregnancy," *Epoch Times*, updated July 20, 2009, www.theepochtimes.com/n2/content/view/18204/.

Birthing Naturally.net, www.birthingnaturally.net/cn/technique/massage.html, www.birthingnaturally.net/cn/technique/knead.html.

"Benefits of Childbirth Meditation," CalmBirth, www.calmbirth.org/benefits.html.

"Meditation during Pregnancy," Yoga Point.com, www.yogapoint.com/info/yogainpregnancy.htm.

"Meditation during Pregnancy," The Intelligence of Soul, mydeepmeditation.com/meditation/benefits-of-meditation/meditation-during-pregnancy/.

"Squatting in Labor," Birthing Naturally, updated September 6, 2011, www.birthingnaturally.net/cn/position/squat.html.

"Slide Show: Labor Positions," Mayo Clinic.com, October 16, 2010, www.mayoclinic.com/health/labor/PR00141.

Jeanne Faulkner, "Breathing Made Easy," *Fit Pregnancy*, October/November 2010, www.fitpregnancy.com/yourpregnancy/labor_delivery/Breathing-Made-Easy-111805199.html.

"Combined Spinal-Epidural (CSE) for Labor Analgesia: The Walking Epidural," Anesthesiology Info.com, 2005, http://anesthesiologyinfo.com/articles/09152002.php.

"Epidural Anesthesia," American Pregnancy Association, last updated August 2007, www.americanpregnancy.org/labornbirth/epidural.html.

"Using Narcotics for Pain Relief during Childbirth," American Pregnancy Association, last updated July 2011, www.americanpregnancy.org/labornbirth/narcotics.html.

CHAPTER 11

"Should You Bank Your Baby's Cord Blood?" *Fit Pregnancy*, Feb/March 2009, www.fitpregnancy.com/baby/health-development/should-you-bank-your-babys-cord-blood.

American Academy of Pediatrics, "Circumcision Policy Statement," *Pediatrics* 103, No. 3 (March 1, 1999), 686–93, http://aappolicy.aappublications.org/cgi/content/full/pediatrics;103/3/686.

Medscape Reference, s.v. "Preclampsia," www.emedicine.medscape.com/article/1476919-overview.

American Congress of Obstetricians and Gynecologists, "ACOG Committee Opinion No. 399: Umbilical Cord Blood Banking," abstract, *Obstetrics & Gynecology* 111, No. 2 (February 2008): 475–77.

"Creating Your Birth Plan," American Pregnancy Association, last updated January, 2012, www.americanpregnancy.org/labornbirth/birthplan.htm.

"Birth Plan Worksheet," Baby Center, http://assets.babycenter.com/ims/Content/birthplan_pdf.pdf.

Katherine Bowers, "The Circumcision Decision," *Fit Pregnancy*, April/May 2010, www.fitpregnancy.com/baby/baby-care/circumcision-decision.

APPENDIX

What to Expect.com Weekly Calendar, www.whattoexpect.com.

Fit Pregnancy, Pregnancy Calendar, www.fitpregnancy.com/calendar.

Babycenter.com, Pregnancy Calendar, www.babycenter.com/pregnancy-calendar.

Babyzone.com, Pregnancy Calendar, www.babyzone.com/pregnancy.

Pregnancy Week by Week, MayoClinic.com, www.mayoclinic.com/health/pregnancy-week-by-week/MY00331

March of Dimes. www.marchofdimes.com/pregnancy/pretermlabor_fetalfibronectin.html.

American Congress of Obstetricians and Gynecologists, *Special Tests for Monitoring Fetal Health*.

ACOG Practice Bulletin, Clinical Management Guidelines for Obstetrician–Gynecologists, Number 55, September 2004.

ACKNOWLEDGMENTS

Thanks to Dana Rousmaniere, my co-writer, for shepherding this book from cover to cover and for being my friend. Thanks to Amanda French and Susan Thomforde for being our inspiring, insightful teammates. Thanks to a few particularly special doctor-buddies who've always provided a wealth of information: Desiree Bley, Janet Gibbens, and Heather Weldon. Thanks to my friends at CARE who've showed me the world that mothers in the developing world live in and how much we can help each other, especially Sarah McCune, Sarah Moser, Ellen Carmichael, and Helene Gayle. Thanks to the many beloved midwives and labor nurses I've worked with through the years who have kept me company through a thousand nightshifts, countless deliveries, and more than enough emergencies. Thanks to my friends and colleagues at *Fit Pregnancy* who supported me through all these years as the "Ask the Labor Nurse" blogger. Thanks to my agent, Kathryn Beaumont, for helping us navigate legal waters and to Cara Connors, our editor. And most of all thanks to my family for absolutely everything.

—JEANNE FAULKNER

Thank you to my co-authors—I couldn't have picked a better team to deliver *this* baby. Thank you for the dedication, knowledge, insights, and experiences that each of you uniquely brought to this book. Thank you to Amanda French and Susan Thomforde for lending your wisdom and expertise. A special thank you to my co-writer, colleague, and friend, Jeanne Faulkner, for laboring along with me through the writing stages of this book, and for making it truly unique. I would also like to thank my former colleagues at *Fit Pregnancy* for four years of insights into pregnancy and birth, and for the opportunity to document two of my own birth experiences for *Fit Pregnancy* readers through my "Charlie Chronicles" and "Baby on Board" blogs. Thank you to our agent, Kathryn Beaumont, for counseling us along the way, as well as our editors at Fair Winds Press, Jill Alexander, Cara Connors, and Betsy Gammons, for their help in bringing this book to fruition. I am most thankful to and for my husband and my family—without you, nothing else matters.

—DANA ROUSMANIERE

ABOUT THE AUTHORS

Amanda V. French, M.D., completed her residency training in obstetrics and gynecology at Boston Medical Center. She is board certified by the American Board of Obstetrics and Gynecology and is a fellow of the American Congress of Obstetrics and Gynecology. She has been employed in private practice with teaching responsibilities at the level of clinical instructor at Brigham and Women's Hospital in Boston. In addition, she has worked as an assistant professor in obstetrics and gynecology at Columbia University Medical Center in New York with the primary responsibility of teaching residents and medical students. Dr. French is now at Boston Children's Hospital and is on the associate staff of Brigham and Women's Hospital in the department of pediatric and adolescent gynecology. Her current academic appointment is Clinical Instructor of Obstetrics, Gynecology, and Reproductive Biology at Harvard Medical School. Dr. French has delivered more than 1,000 babies over the course of her career. She considers herself lucky and blessed to have had two uncomplicated pregnancies and births, and is the proud mother of two sons.

Susan Thomforde, C.N.M., has been a practicing nurse midwife for more than twenty-seven years. She's been called "a midwife's midwife"—the highest compliment in midwifery. She was a member of the Tufts University faculty while working at St. Margaret's Hospital and has been an adjunct faculty member for Yale University, Case Western Reserve University, and University of Pennsylvania midwifery students. For the past seventeen years, she's been delivering babies at the North Shore Birth Center in Beverly, Massachusetts—one of two free-standing birth centers in Massachusetts. Susan was inspired to be a midwife by her aunt, who was one of the early nurse midwives in the United States in the 1930s. She has delivered more than 1,000 babies—and three children of her own—with her sister midwives. When she's not working, Susan spends time knitting and working in her garden.

ABOUT THE AUTHORS

Jeanne Faulkner, R.N., has a twenty-year history as a labor and delivery, postpartum, neonatal, and NICU nurse and a ten-year history as a health writer. She studied nursing at Los Angeles County–USC Medical Center School of Nursing and California State University, Los Angeles. She's helped thousands of parents through every possible birthing scenario from the most natural to the most complicated. She shares her real-world perspective and practical advice on the obstacles and opportunities parents face both inside and outside the hospital in her weekly column for *Fit Pregnancy* magazine online called "Ask the Labor Nurse," and contributes regularly to *Fit Pregnancy* magazine, the *Oregonian* newspaper, the *Huffington Post*, www.QualityHealth.com, and www.MyRegence.com. Her work has appeared in *Better Homes and Gardens*, *Real Simple*, *Shape*, *Northwest Healthy Living*, and many other publications and websites. Jeanne's kids range in age from middle-school to mid-20s, via four vaginal deliveries, three epidurals, and one out-of-hospital, natural birth in her midwife's office. She's also an advocate, writer, speaker, and lobbyist for global women's and maternal health issues and has traveled with CARE (a global humanitarian organization) to work with mothers around the world.

Dana Rousmaniere is a writer, editor, and author who has written for print and online publications, including *Good Housekeeping*, *Healthy Living*, *Living Fit*, *Women's Health*, the *Atlantic Monthly Online*, Babble.com, CafeMom.com, and more. She was managing editor of *Fit Pregnancy* magazine online for many years, and has also held positions as senior producer at Lifetime Television Online and new media editor for Hearst Publishing. Her *Fit Pregnancy* blog, the Charlie Chronicles, was a finalist for the 2007 Maggie Awards for Best Regularly Featured Web Column. She is also the author of *North Shore Baby*, a field guide for Boston-area parents. Dana delivered two of her babies in the hospital with epidurals, and delivered her third child—a 10.5 pound baby!—in a drug-free water birth. She lives with her husband and three children on the North Shore of Massachusetts.

PHOTOGRAPHER CREDITS

INDEX